# CARDIOVASCULAR PHYSIOLOGY IN EXERCISE AND SPORT

THE UNIVERSITY OF
WINCHESTER

D1471039

## Publisher's Note

The author, Professor Christopher Bell, sadly died during production of this book. Dr. Stuart Warmington was nominated by Professor Bell to carry out the final checking of proofs and we thank him for this work.

For Elsevier:

Commissioning Editor: Claire Wilson
Development Editor: Catherine Jackson
Project Manager: Andrew Palfreyman
Designer: Charlotte Murray
Illustrations Manager: Merlyn Harvey
Illustrator: Joanna Cameron

# CARDIOVASCULAR PHYSIOLOGY IN EXERCISE AND SPORT

## Christopher Bell

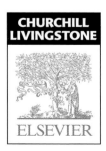

CHURCHILL
LIVINGSTONE

ELSEVIER

EDINBURGH LONDON NEW YORK OXFORD PHILADELPHIA ST LOUIS SYDNEY TORONTO 2008

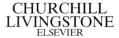

# CHURCHILL LIVINGSTONE
## ELSEVIER

First published 2008
ISBN: 978 0 443 06965 9

**British Library Cataloguing in Publication Data**
A catalogue record for this book is available from the British Library.

**Library of Congress Cataloging in Publication Data**
A catalog record for this book is available from the Library of Congress.

**Note**
Knowledge and best practice in this field are constantly changing. As new research and experience broaden our knowledge, changes in practice, treatment and drug therapy may become necessary or appropriate. Readers are advised to check the most current information provided (i) on procedures featured or (ii) by the manufacturer of each product to be administered, to verify the recommended dose or formula, the method and duration of administration, and contraindications. It is the responsibility of the practitioner, relying on their own experience and knowledge of the patient, to make diagnoses, to determine dosages and the best treatment for each individual patient, and to take all appropriate safety precautions. To the fullest extent of the law, neither the Publisher nor the Author assumes any liability for any injury and/or damage to persons or property arising out or related to any use of the material contained in this book.

The Publisher

Printed in China

The publisher's policy is to use **paper manufactured from sustainable forests**

II

# CONTENTS

# PREFACE

Exercise – *'labour of the body: considered as conducive to the cure or prevention of diseases.'*

Samuel Johnson (1755)

At universities around the world, large numbers of students are studying human physiology in programmes leading to degrees in natural sciences or exercise science. Many will go on to professional careers in sports medicine, cardiac rehabilitation, exercise science or academic human physiology. These students require a different level of understanding of cardiovascular function to that needed for students of medicine and other health sciences. In particular, they require solid foundation knowledge on how the cardiovascular system responds and adapts to exercise and to the associated environmental challenges, together with practical information on how various parameters of circulatory function can be measured in real life, by the practising physiologist. That is my purpose in this book.

It is equally important to make it clear at the outset what is NOT the purpose of the book. First, it is written for advanced students who have dealt already with the basic principles of cardiovascular function in earlier courses, so a certain level of basic understanding is expected. Second, I have not tried to cover all aspects of advanced cardiovascular physiology. There are several excellent and scholarly books of this type already on the market – for example, Rowell (1993), Levick (2003), Klabunde (2004), Berne & Levy (2001) and Noble et al (2005) – and another would not contribute anything new. Finally, this book is most definitely not intended as a comprehensive manual of strategies for optimizing physical performance. These practical issues are covered at an appropriate level for most readers in several textbooks of exercise and sports physiology and in more depth in a comprehensive publication from the American Council of Sports Medicine (American Council of Sports Medicine 2005).

Nonetheless, there is of course a certain degree of overlap in content and emphasis with these other categories of book, and both might be used to supplement and reinforce the material that appears here. For example, most textbooks of exercise physiology contain abundant diagrams illustrating the circulatory adjustments to different exercise paradigms and so I have not attempted to replicate these. To my mind, Plowman & Smith (2003) is especially useful from this point of view. If you are able to access it, I also recommend viewing a film produced by Sandoz some years ago entitled *Blood Pressure Telemetry*. This provides a unique opportunity of seeing moment-by-moment cardiovascular responses to exercise and other stresses in unrestrained human volunteers.

Each chapter of *Cardiovascular Physiology in Exercise and Sport* begins with a statement of the main learning objectives. Each ends with a summary of the most important points covered, some revision questions and a list of further reading for students who wish to explore aspects of the area in more depth. I have not provided exhaustive reference lists, which are in my opinion not particularly useful in a student text and are, in any case, redundant when virtually every reader has access to electronic bibliographic services. The text is accompanied by boxed Case histories that illustrate real-life scenarios, boxed summaries of common practical procedures and diagrams that are unique to this book and that I believe help understanding of areas that are often difficult for the student. In addition, to the rear of the book are a series of multiple-choice questions linking back to each chapter.

It is inevitable that a book that discusses quantitative human function will contain numerous numerical values. The absolute values of many parameters may be very different in different populations and I have tried to indicate how physical characteristics affect each parameter. For consistency, however, I have generally used baseline values that reflect the body of international research data. This means that they are what might be expected for young male adults weighing around 70 kg, and who are of Caucasian origin. Any reader who feels disenfranchized by this may take comfort in the knowledge that generating reliable values for other ethnic groups would be a very valuable project.

This book would probably have never been written were it not for the feedback from many students over the years and I should like to record my thanks for their input. I hope that you, the reader, find it a useful learning resource. Best wishes for your career in human physiology.

Christopher Bell
Dublin, 2007

## References

American College of Sports Medicine 2005 Advanced Exercise Physiology. Lippincott Williams & Wilkins, Philadephia.

Berne RM, Levy MN 2001 Cardiovascular Physiology, 8th edn. Mosby, St Louis.

Klabunde RF 2004 Cardiovascular Physiology Concepts. Lippincott, Philadelphia.

Levick JR 2003 Introduction to Cardiovascular Physiology, 4th edn. Arnold, London.

Noble A, Johnson RA, Thomas A, Bass P 2005 The Cardiovascular System. Churchill Livingstone, Edinburgh.

Plowman SA, Smith D 2003 Exercise Physiology for Health, Fitness and Performance, 2nd edn. Benjamin Cummings, San Francisco.

Rowell LB 1993 Human Cardiovascular Control. OUP, Oxford.

# ACKNOWLEDGEMENTS

I am grateful to Professor Michael Walsh for providing the data shown in Figures 2.2, 2.3 and 2.4, Dr Saoirse O'Sullivan for the data shown in Figure 2.5, Ms Áine Murray for the data shown in Figures 4.2, 7.1 and 11.1 and Dr Maeve Barry for the data shown in Figure 7.2.

Several colleagues with a range of expertise in exercise physiology and sports science have read sections of the manuscript in various stages of its preparation and I thank them all for their comments and suggestions. I am particularly grateful to Professor Mark Hargeaves (University of Melbourne), Professor Ian MacDonald, Dr Soairse O'Sullivan (both University of Nottingham) and Dr Stuart Warmington (University of Dublin) for having read and commented on the final draft. All the defects that remain are of my own making.

## Chapter 1

# Introduction: the whole–body response to exercise

**After reading this chapter, you should:**

- appreciate that absolute work capacity is ultimately limited by cardiovascular performance
- understand the overall cardiovascular changes that occur during exercise
- be ready to track the mechanisms that underlie these changes through the succeeding chapters.

The basic pattern of cardiovascular response to acute exercise is straightforward. It is centred on the principle that the cardiovascular system fulfils three primary functions: to deliver nutrients and oxygen to cells of the body's tissues, to remove metabolites from the same sites and to regulate heat exchange between body and environment so as to maintain a stable core temperature. It is self-evident that increased metabolic activity in skeletal muscles must require increased local blood flow and that this metabolic activity must produce heat that needs to be dissipated.

Ultimately, the absolute amount of work that an individual can perform depends on the capacity of the circulation to service muscle metabolism and to maintain thermal stability. The efficiency of muscle cell contraction can of course affect exercise performance and the time to fatigue, so factors such as the cellular concentrations of mitochondria and myoglobin must be taken into account. If we compare trained and sedentary subjects, then the difference in work capacity will be partly due to the adaptive effects of training on muscle cell metabolism. However, no degree of muscular adaptation can enhance aerobic performance unless there is concomitant cardiovascular adaptation and, in highly trained individuals, this increased capacity for aerobic activity is limited entirely by blood flow. Similarly, despite the multiple factors that contribute to fatigue, it is the encroachment on circulatory performance that has the most predictable and the most potentially serious consequences.

The amount of skeletal muscle activation that occurs during exercise must by definition be proportional to the activity of descending neural instructions from the cerebral motor cortex. This offers an ideal way by which circulatory responses can be regulated in proportion to the extent of motor activity, via collateral inputs from the descending motor axons onto the hindbrain nuclei that control the sympathetic nervous system. These inputs activate sympathetic outflows to the heart and peripheral blood vessels, increasing cardiac output and blood pressure. At the same time, a combination of local mechanisms in the microcirculation of the active muscles ensures that these vessels are relaxed so that the elevated cardiac and perfusion pressure gradient result in increased muscle blood flow. This situation is summarized, in its simplest form, in Figure 1.1 below.

The next few chapters will be concerned with the mechanisms by which these basic events take place, together with some of the practicalities of measuring them in human subjects. We shall progressively expand upon the flow diagram shown in Figure 1.1, aiming to finish up with a complete diagrammatic description of the interactions that occur during acute exercise. We shall then examine the ways in which circulatory efficiency limits exercise in different circumstances and some of the factors that can curtail exercise by interfering with circulatory function. Finally, we shall look at the ways in which cardiovascular adaptation to chronic exercise improves the efficiency of the acute exercise response, and how this adaptation is affected by exposure to different altitudes.

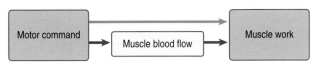

**Figure 1.1** Basics of the relationships between motor command of exercise and the associated muscle work and muscle blood flow.

# Chapter 2

# Cardiac activation

## CHAPTER CONTENTS

### After reading this chapter, you should:

- understand the functional characteristics that allow the heart to operate efficiently at rest and during exercise
- appreciate how the electrocardiogram can be used to obtain information on the normal heart
- be able to recognize the main cardiac arrhythmias that are likely exclusion criteria for participation in exercise programmes.

## REQUIREMENTS FOR AN EFFECTIVE HEART

As a foundation from which to explore the responses of the circulation to exercise and environment, it is worthwhile to review the characteristics that the heart requires in order to fulfil its role as a pump. At least most of the material covered in this first section is probably familiar to you from earlier courses, but it may be helpful to have it set out again. As you read through the first section of this chapter, use the simulated records in Figure 2.1 to remind yourself of the sequences of electrical and mechanical events that make up the cardiac cycle.

### Rhythmic excitation

For a muscular pump to provide continuous blood flow through the circulation there must be a system that guarantees generation of muscle action

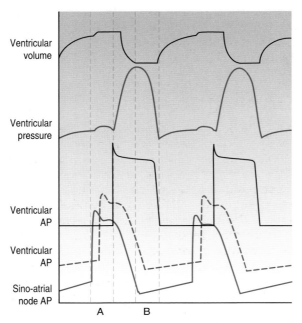

**Figure 2.1** Relative timecourses of electrical and mechanical events during the cardiac cycle. Note the long time delays between electrical activation of the sinoatrial node and arrival of an action potential in the ventricular muscle (A), and between the beginning and end of ventricular repolarization (B).

potentials at regular intervals. The normal rhythm generator or pacemaker is a small group of cells that lies high in the wall of the right atrium, constituting the so-called *sinoatrial node*. The membranes of these cells have an unusually high sodium conductance and contain metabolic pumps that progressively reduce potassium conductance. These two properties together result in the membrane potential depolarizing gradually towards zero in what is termed the *pacemaker potential*, rather than them having a stable resting membrane potential of around −70 mV as is characteristic of the normal cardiac muscle cells. Since the threshold membrane potential for action potential initiation is around −40 mV, the pacemaker cells fire an action potential as soon as they depolarize to this threshold. As in any excitable cell, the action potential activates a delayed potassium efflux and this repolarizes the cells to around −70 mV but, once these voltage-gated potassium channels close, the membrane starts to depolarize once more and initiates another action potential.

The period between successive action potentials in a sinoatrial node cell at 37° C (98.5° F) is around 600 ms, giving an inherent frequency of cardiac excitation of about 100 beats/min. In the intact body, however, the slope of the pacemaker potential is subject to tonic influences by thoracic sympathetic nerves that increase the slope and speed up heart rate (*tachycardia*) and vagal parasympathetic nerves that reduce the slope and slow the heart down (*bradycardia*). In a resting subject, both of these neural inputs are continuously active but the bradycardic effect of the parasympathetic input predominates, so that resting heart rate is normally less than 100 beats/min and typically around 65–75 beats/min.

## Duration of pressurization

It takes only about 50 ms to pressurize the blood contained within the cardiac chambers, but physical movement of that blood out into the arterial system takes several times longer and so ventricular compression needs to be maintained for much longer than in other types of muscle cell. This maintained pressurization is due to the presence of slow voltage-gated calcium channels whose opening follows the fast sodium-dependent rising phase of the action potential and which remain open for several hundred ms. Inward movement of calcium through these channels produces the characteristic plateau phase of the cardiac action potential. The calcium channel cycle time and the action potential plateau phase are shorter in atrial than in ventricular muscle cells, reflecting the fact that ejection from the ventricles has to overcome a greater downstream resistance than that faced by the atria and so movement of the same volume of fluid takes longer.

## Delay between atrial and ventricular activation

For impulses from the sino-atrial node to produce synchronized contractions of the whole heart, the cardiac myocytes need to be coupled into an electrical syncytium. The position of the sinoatrial node within the atria means that action potential spread necessarily activates the atrial muscle first and only then gains access to the ventricles. This provides the correct sequence required for pumping of blood from atria to ventricles, but a single syncytium encompassing atria and ventricles would be impracticable, since ventricular pressurization would begin almost immediately after atrial contraction, allowing insufficient time for ventricular filling to be completed. Instead, the syncytium of the atria and the syncytium of the ventricles are separated by an insulative layer of connective tissue, with electrical continuity between atria and ventricles only via the specialized cells of the *atrioventricular (A/V) node*. These cells are very small in diameter and, therefore, conduct action potentials very slowly, conferring a delay of 120–200 ms between the beginning of atrial muscle depolarization and the arrival of action potentials in the ventricular muscle.

## Direction of ventricular pressure gradient

The ventricular chambers are elongated, with the outlets into the arterial system lying at their rostral ends adjacent to the A/V margin. Efficient blood ejection, therefore, requires progressive development of pressure from the ventricular apex towards the exit site, although the apical region is furthest away from the point of entry of action potentials through the A/V node. To achieve the appropriate sequence of ventricular activation, the ventricular end of the A/V node is connected to a branching system of large-diameter (that is, fast-conducting) cells forming the *Purkinje system*. This conducting system travels down each side of the interventricular septum, bypassing the more rostral regions of the ventricular muscle and directing excitation directly to the endocardial surface of the ventricular apices. Excitation then propagates back through the syncytium towards the A/V margin, pushing the ventricular contents towards its arterial exit points. The efficiency of ejection is further enhanced by the fact that the muscle making up the outer ventricular walls is arranged spirally, so that when it contracts it produces a wringing movement.

## Guaranteed time for filling

After ventricular contraction finishes and the heart relaxes, there must be time for the ventricles to relax completely so that they can refill. Thus, a safety mechanism must exist to guard against another action potential causing re-excitation while some muscle cells are still contracted. To achieve this the voltage-gated calcium channels in the endocardial muscle cells nearest to the conducting system have longer cycle times than those in the more superficial muscle layers, with correspondingly longer plateau phases and refractory periods. Thus, the cells that are coupled to the Purkinje system will remain electrically non-excitable until the rest of the ventricular muscle has repolarized and relaxed. The difference in channel cycle time between endocardium and epicardium is due at least partly to the higher pressure that is exerted on membranes of the endocardial cells when the heart wall contracts.

An additional safety factor is that the action potential plateau of the Purkinje fibres themselves is significantly longer than that of any ventricular myocardial cell, so that a second impulse is unlikely even to reach the ventricular myocardium until this has relaxed entirely.

Existence of a finite relaxation period is a prerequisite for nutritional perfusion of the ventricular myocardium. The coronary arteries that supply the heart arise from the aorta and so the pressure gradient responsible for coronary blood flow is essentially identical to that generated by the left ventricle. Because ventricular ejection must involve at least equivalent pressure being developed within the left ventricular wall, the left coronary arteries are mechanically occluded during the ejection phase of the cardiac cycle (termed *systole*) and nutritional perfusion can occur only during the relaxation phase (termed *diastole*). As will be discussed in Chapter 8 (p. 95), coronary perfusion of the right ventricle is more continuous, since the ventricular pressure developed there is much lower than systemic arterial pressure, and so the vasculature is perfused during systole as well as diastole.

## Coordination of right and left outputs

Since the systemic and pulmonary circulations are in series, they must each pump identical volumes of blood per unit time. It is, therefore, essential that both ventricles eject blood simultaneously. This coordinated timing is ensured by the fact that the Purkinje system conveys action potentials simultaneously to the apices of both ventricles. Even with exact timing, however, the left ventricle needs to generate a far greater ejection pressure than the right ventricle in order to eject the same volume of blood, because the systemic vasculature has a much higher resistance than does the pulmonary vasculature. To provide the extra degree of pressurization, the left ventricle is wrapped with an additional spiral layer of muscle.

Increased venous return, for example in response to lying down, will produce a corresponding rise in end-diastolic ventricular volume. If the volume of blood ejected with each systolic contraction (the *stroke volume*) remained constant, there would be progressive pooling of blood in the heart and a progressive fall in cardiac output, so it is important that stroke volume can be matched automatically to ventricular filling. This is achieved by the resting length of all ventricular muscle fibres being substantially below the length that would correspond to optimal actin/myosin crossbridging and development of maximal active shortening. With increased filling, the increased resting sarcomere length that results from passive stretch of the ventricular wall will therefore result in increased active tension. This phenomenon is known as the *Frank-Starling relationship*.

## MONITORING ELECTRICAL ACTIVITY OF THE HEART

## Basis of the electrocardiogram

### Timecourses and amplitudes of events

When voltage is recorded between two points in an excitable tissue, the electrode towards which a wave of membrane depolarization is moving becomes positive relative to the other electrode, while a wave of repolarization causes the reverse voltage difference. During excitation of the heart, the sequence of electrical events is highly predictable. Continual measurement of voltage difference across the heart can, therefore, be used to identify the timing of depolarization of atria and ventricles, while the magnitude of voltage changes indicates the volume of muscle that is involved. The characteristic voltage record obtained is termed the *electrocardiogram*, or ECG, and the sequence of electrical events that occurs during cardiac excitation can be tracked by identifying each of the phases of the ECG waveform with a specific letter (Fig. 2.2).

With normal excitation originating from the sinoatrial node, measurement of the time between the beginning of atrial depolarization (beginning of P wave) and the entry of action potentials into the muscle of the ventricular apices (beginning of R wave) is always between 120 and 200 ms. Most of this delay

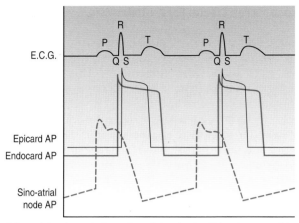

**Figure 2.2** Timing of sinoatrial and ventricular endocardial and epicardial action potentials, relative to the ECG.

is due to action potential travel through the slowly conducting A/V pathway, producing the so-called *P–R interval* which provides an index of the efficiency of this path. Ventricular excitation occurs by simultaneous entry of action potentials into both apices and coordinated spread of depolarization over both ventricles. This process takes only 60–80 ms and is indicated by the duration of the QRS complex. Once ventricular depolarization is complete the muscle cells all remain depolarized for the duration of the action potential plateau and then progressively repolarize, producing the T wave. This sequence produces an initial isoelectric period typically around 150 ms in duration while all cells are depolarized, and then a T wave whose timecourse of around 200 ms represents the range of action potential durations in different regions of the ventricular wall.

Since the endocardial cells have longer plateau durations than the epicardial cells, the sequence of repolarization between the different muscle layers is in the reverse order to the sequence of depolarization. For this reason, the voltage polarity of the T wave is usually the same as that of the R wave. In hearts with hypertrophied ventricles, however, greater epicardial intramural pressure is produced during contraction and the differences in plateau duration between epicardial and endocardial regions are reduced. As a result the ventricular cells tend to repolarize in the same sequence as they depolarized, producing an inverted T wave.

## Orientations of ECG recording

The voltage changes occurring across the heart spread without diminution throughout the highly conductive medium of the body interior and can be detected from the body surface, so long as electrolyte-rich liquid is rubbed into the skin under the recording electrodes in order to overcome the high electrical resistance of the epidermis. Recording can be made most simply between right and left arms (Lead II) or between one arm and the left leg (Leads I and III). This so-called *frontal lead* system allows detection of impulse movement across the heart either horizontally or in a semi-vertical direction. Usually, the primary concerns for human physiologists are simply to have a signal large enough for you to be certain whether or not the sequence of excitation is normal, and to be able to reliably trigger a ratemeter from the R wave. Lead II usually provides the best record for these purposes but, because different people's hearts have different vertical-horizontal orientations, larger signals are seen with one of the other lead orientations in some individuals.

## HANDY HINTS

Although the frontal lead system is usually referred to as using arms and legs, the only criterion for placement of electrodes is that they should be outside the limits of the heart. During exercise, contraction of superficial muscles underneath an electrode can produce a voltage deflection that looks something like a QRS complex. Therefore, when movement patterns involve activation of arm muscle, positioning the electrodes on wrists or arms sometimes leads to apparently abnormal records (Chatterjee 2006). For this reason, it is best practice in studies involving limb movement to place the electrodes on the chest wall or shoulders.

Because there is little arm movement, cleaner ECG signals are seen during cycle ergometry than during treadmill running, but at high work intensities mechanical interference from muscle activity often makes it impossible to obtain consistent records regardless of the type of exercise. In addition, the high rate of sweating with heavy exercise makes self-adhesive electrodes fall off. If the sole purpose of the ECG is to monitor heart rate, then the best solution is to use a thoracic belt and telemetric monitoring of R wave frequency using a Polar$^{TM}$ watch or similar device.

Electrical activity moving at right angles to the orientation of the ECG electrodes produces no voltage signal, so frontal leads provide only limited information on the three-dimensional spread of activity through the heart. For this purpose, it is necessary to also record voltage differences between the heart and different points along the ventrodorsal diameter of the chest. The standard points used are six locations ranging from the right side of the sternum overlying the right ventricle (Lead $V_1$), to the left axilla overlying the left ventricle (Lead $V_6$). With these leads, one would expect to see a positive R wave in $V_6$, but a reversed R wave in $V_1$ reflecting the relative muscle masses in the two ventricles. So it is not surprising that at one or two of the intermediate locations, where the recording electrodes overlie the interventricular septum, the R wave appears bipolar. The chest leads are particularly useful for recognizing changes in absolute muscle volume in one or other ventricle, which alters the pattern of R wave polarity between the six locations. In addition, the R wave in $V_6$ is the largest in amplitude of any lead but never normally exceeds 2.5 mV. An R wave from this lead that is 3 mV or more in height can, therefore, be used as a reliable index of left ventricular hypertrophy, and constitutes one of the indices for assessing training-induced cardiovascular adaptation in athletes (see Chapter 11, p. 131).

## Arrhythmias in the normal heart

The term *arrhythmia* refers to any deviation of heart rate from a steady value between the limits of 60–100 beats/min. So, strictly speaking, heart rate is arrhythmic whenever it fluctuates or is outside the 60–100 beats/min range. Despite its popular connotations, therefore, arrhythmia does not necessarily imply abnormal cardiac function.

### Effects of local temperature

The membrane events that determine the slope of the pacemaker potential in sinoatrial cells depend on metabolic pumps and all metabolic processes are temperature-dependent. Therefore, changes in deep body temperature will affect heart rate by a direct effect on sinoatrial discharge frequency, with a rise in blood temperature of 0.5°C increasing heart rate by about 8 beats/min. It is not possible to know how much this process affects the efficiency of cardiac output changes in response to exercise or to hot environments, but it has to be considered when evaluating the absolute magnitude of tachycardia that occurs under these conditions.

### Exercise tachycardia

The descending pathways that travel from motor cortex to spinal motor neurons and produce muscle movement also provide inputs to the cardiovascular control centre in the hindbrain, inhibiting vagal and increasing sympathetic drive to the sinoatrial node. Thus, heart rate increases proportionately to exercise intensity, with even very low workloads producing heart rates of above 100 beats/min.

At heart rates of 150 beats/min or higher, successive T and P waves follow each other without time for any isoelectric period. The absence of an isoelectric period makes the record look as if there is some irregularity of excitation (Fig. 2.3A). However, inspection will confirm that there is a regular sequence of P, QRS and T waves.

### Training bradycardia

Chronic aerobic activity results in a progressive fall in resting heart rate. With moderate activity the reduction is typically only 5–10 beats/min and occurs over several weeks' activity. With the more intense levels of training

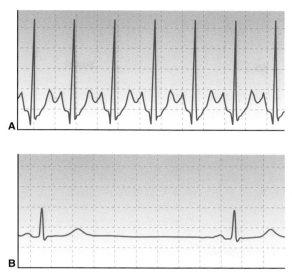

**Figure 2.3** Typical ECG records from normal subjects near the extremes of the heart rate range. As in all ECG recordings, each large grid square represents 200 ms and 0.5 mV. In (A) the subject is exercising and heart rate is once every 400 ms or 150 beats/min. Note the loss of an isoelectric interval between T and P waves, but the maintenance of a stable P–R interval of just under 200 ms and a regular sequence of P, QRS and T waves. (B) This shows a heart rate of 35 beats/min in a highly trained athlete at rest. Note that the P–R interval is still less than 200 ms. These two records also show the considerable shortening of the ventricular action potential with increased heart rate, as measured by the time between the R and T waves.

associated with competitive aerobic exercise, resting rate continues to fall to values that may be as low as 30–35 beats/min in elite athletes. The mechanisms that underlie this progressive training bradycardia will be examined in Chapter 11 (p. 133). As with exercise tachycardia, extreme bradycardia makes the ECG record look strange (Fig. 2.3B). However, its normality can be confirmed easily by checking that the PR interval is normal and that there is a consistent sequence of P, R and T waves. Note that, without an ECG, it would be impossible to know whether somebody with a very slow heart rate is a normal, athletically fit person or has some cardiac abnormality that slows down the heart beat.

*Respiratory sinus arrhythmia*

Heart rate shows a sinusoidal oscillation during the respiratory cycle, with a relative tachycardia developing during inspiration and waning during expiration. This oscillation is due to the fact that vagal drive to the sinoatrial node falls progressively as inspiration progresses. Two inhibitory inputs to the vagal centre in the hindbrain are involved, one from stretch receptors in the lung and one from inspiratory neurons in the hindbrain respiratory centre. As the discharges of both these inhibitory pathways are proportional to the amount of inspiratory effort, the magnitude of sinus arrhythmia is much greater during deep than shallow breathing. Even at rest, however, there is typically a variation of at least 5–10 beats/min in individuals below the age of 30. A representative example of sinus arrhythmia can be seen in Figure 4.3 (p. 37).

By middle age, little or no heart rate variability is seen except during deep breathing and with further ageing the variability disappears altogether. This decline is not due to alteration in resting vagal tone (since resting heart rate does not change substantially with age), but probably involves changes in gain of the central input pathways to the vagal centre. Damage to the vagus is a common early component of peripheral nerve degeneration in patients with type I diabetes and, therefore, the magnitude of sinus arrhythmia in younger diabetics is a useful index in assessing their clinical status.

The bradycardia that results from chronic physical training is accompanied by increased magnitude of sinus arrhythmia, probably reflecting the increased range over which altered vagal tone can alter heart rate. In fact, the absolute magnitude of the arrhythmia has been suggested to provide a quantitative index of fitness, similar to that derived from measurement of $\dot{V}O_{2max}$ (Lopes & White 2006).

## Abnormal arrhythmias

Damage from altered plasma electrolyte levels, from inadequate local blood flow (*ischaemia*) or from local trauma can affect pacemaker function, integrity of the cardiac conducting system or membrane excitability and any of these changes will be reflected in the ECG pattern. Detailed clinical assessment of ECGs is the responsibility of a cardiologist, but all physiologists who are involved with human subjects should be able to spot the most obvious abnormal arrhythmias so that they can decide whether a subject should be excluded from a programme that involves added cardiovascular demand. A good-quality 12-lead ECG record will allow the following abnormal patterns to be identified.

### Absence of P waves

Normal atrial muscle can only be activated once by a single sinoatrial impulse, because the prolonged plateau phase of the atrial action potential maintains it in a refractory state. If, however, the conduction velocity of the action potential is slowed by local hypoxia, or the distance needed for the action potential to travel around the atrial wall is increased because the atria have been stretched, or the action potential plateau phase duration is reduced by altered channel cycling, then a single action potential may circulate through the tissue over and over again and cause repetitive but uncoordinated contractions. This phenomenon is termed *atrial fibrillation*.

Atrial fibrillation has relatively little effect on the efficiency of cardiac pumping because most ventricular filling has occurred before atrial systole (Fig. 2.1). But it does create a potential problem. Instead of the atrial contents being regularly ejected, some blood tends to lie stationary in the extremities of the atrial chambers. When blood is stagnant, it tends to form clots and cell aggregates (*thrombi*) (see also Chapter 5, p. 48). If these thrombi are mobilized into the cardiac output, for instance during the vigorous respiratory effort of exercise, then they may occlude vessels in the coronary or cerebral circulation, causing a heart attack or stroke. Individuals with evidence of atrial fibrillation should, therefore, not be recruited into exercise programmes without careful clinical assessment.

Atrial fibrillation can be identified by two characteristics. First, no P wave exists because the action potentials that spread through the atria do not all travel in the same direction and so do not produce a reproducible voltage deflection on the ECG trace. Second, heart rate varies widely from beat to beat, in an unpredictable pattern (Fig. 2.4). This is because the disorganized direction of action potential travel means that they arrive at the A/V node at irregular intervals, with some arriving while the node cells are still in their refractory period from the previous action potential. In all other arrhythmias that involve varying heart rate there is either a progressive rise and fall in frequency (see Sinus arrhythmia, above) or intermittent insertion of extra R waves into an otherwise regular sequence (see Ventricular extrasystole, below).

### Abnormal relationship between P and R waves

Damage to the cells of the A/V node may occur due to local ischaemia, inflammation, physical pressure by scar tissue or local calcification. This can have either of two separate effects on impulse conduction. In some cases there is slowing of action potential propagation with prolongation of the P–R interval beyond the normal upper limit of 200 ms, typically to 300–400 ms (Fig. 2.5A). In other cases, the effect of the damage is not to slow conduction velocity, but instead to slow calcium channel cycle time, so that following passage of one action potential the node is still refractory when the next impulse arrives. As a result, only every second or third action potential

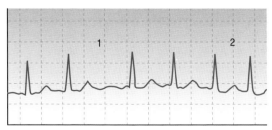

**Figure 2.4** ECG recording from a patient with atrial fibrillation. As in all ECG recordings, each large grid square represents 200 ms and 0.5 mV. The relationship between R and T waves is normal, but no P waves exist and heart rate varies dramatically from beat to beat, between about 100 beats/min (1) and 190 beats/min (2). Note that when heart rate is high, it is essential to identify the matching of R to T waves in order to avoid misinterpreting T waves as P waves.

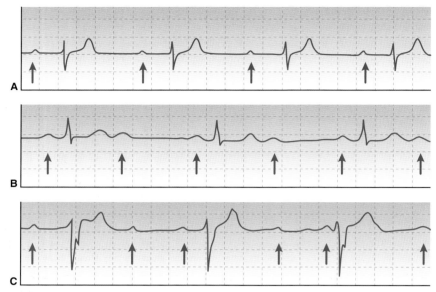

**Figure 2.5** ECG records demonstrating different degrees of atrioventricular block. As in all ECG recordings, each large grid square represents 200 ms and 0.5 mV. (A) First degree block. Every P wave (arrowed) is associated with ventricular excitation but the P–R interval is prolonged – here to around 360 ms. (B) Second degree block. Only every second P wave (arrowed) causes ventricular excitation. Note the consistent duration of the P–R interval in these cycles. (C) Third degree (complete) block. In contrast with (B), there is no consistent time linkage of P and R waves. The identifiable P waves are arrowed, but the irregular rhythm indicates that there are additional events masked by the T waves, giving a true atrial excitation rate of around once every 500 ms (120/min).

enters the ventricle and the ECG shows QRS complexes and T waves associated only with every second or third P wave (Fig. 2.5B).

If the nodal cells are damaged severely enough then they are unable to propagate impulses at all, and ventricles and atria become electrically insulated from each other. Although the sinoatrial node continues to discharge and, therefore, P waves occur at their normal frequency, ventricular activation can originate only from within the ventricular system. The intraventricular Purkinje system contains a number of cells that have similar membrane properties to those of the sinoatrial cells but depolarize much more slowly. These cells normally never reach action potential threshold before they are activated by an impulse arriving from the A/V node. When this is prevented, however, these slower pacemakers can take over control of ventricular rhythm with frequencies in the range of 30–45 beats/min. The result is QRS complexes and T waves at a much lower frequency than that of the P waves and with no consistent association between P and R waves (Fig. 2.5C).

Clearly, lack of synchrony between atrial and ventricular pumping frequency denotes a heart that is not likely to be able to accommodate efficiently to demands for increased output. Individuals in whom you suspect

A/V block should, therefore, not be recruited into exercise programmes without referral to a cardiologist.

### Abnormal QRS complexes

Normally, action potentials travel from the A/V node down the Purkinje fibres on left and right sides of the interventricular septum. This produces simultaneous depolarization of both ventricles, with a QRS complex that is never more than 80 ms in duration. The synchronization of ventricular depolarization can be disrupted by damage to one of the branches of the Purkinje system, so that one ventricle is activated before the other. Alternatively, arrival of impulses through the conducting system may be normal, but an area of ventricular muscle may be damaged (usually by ischaemia) so that the sequence of spread of action potentials through the ventricular syncytium is disrupted. Any of these changes will result in a longer period being taken for ventricular depolarization, with concomitant widening of the QRS complex and usually some loss of the sharp 'spikiness' of the R wave.

Sometimes in a normal heart, the membrane of a cell within the ventricular Purkinje system or the ventricular muscle becomes hyperexcitable and generates an action potential. This causes an additional QRS complex and an extra ventricular contraction. Such a so-called *extrasystole* can be distinguished by two characteristics. First, the fact that it originates from a site distal to the Purkinje system means that activation of the myocardium follows a different route to normal, producing a QRS complex that has a different shape and is longer in duration. Second, the action potential plateau produces a refractory state in the myocardial cells that prevents activation by the next normal action potential, so an extrasystole is followed by a longer than normal pause before the next contraction. This is termed a *compensatory pause*.

## Case history

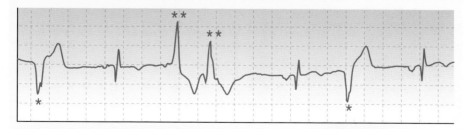

Brian K, a sedentary male, heavy smoker, 50 years old, volunteered for an exercise training study. His ECG was recorded at rest and part of the record is shown above.

# Discussion

Interspersed with normal ECG waveforms, this record showed frequent R waves that were followed by T waves but were not preceded by P waves. The prolonged duration of these R waves and the fact that they were dissimilar in shape to those in the normal beats indicates that they originated from the ventricular musculature. More important, however, was the danger sign that they were of two different shapes and polarities (marked * and **), indicating that they arose from two quite different areas of the ventricular syncytium. This is often a warning of poor coronary perfusion. Brian was advised that he could not be admitted safely into the training programme and was referred to a cardiology clinic.

Extrasystoles are relatively common, especially in individuals who are overtired, stressed or have ingested caffeine. When every extrasystolic QRS has the same shape and timecourse they do not signify any pathology and do not interfere with exercise, since they disappear as soon as heart rate begins to increase. By contrast, you may see extrasystolic QRS complexes that vary in shape from one to the other, indicating that they are initiated from more than one region of the ventricular muscle (see Case history). This pattern is seen most usually in smokers and is suggestive of a poor coronary blood supply. People exhibiting these multifocal extrasystoles should never be enrolled in an exercise programme without prior screening by a cardiologist.

## Key points

The ability of the heart to function as a mechanical pump depends not only on its capacity to develop contractile force, but also on the timing of contraction in different parts of the heart.

The ECG provides an easy way of checking the sequence of timing.

Abnormal aspects of timing that need to be considered in subjects being admitted to exercise programmes are lack of organized atrial contraction, lack of communication between atria and ventricles, and presence of extra ventricular contractions.

## References

Chatterjee D 2006 A shaky moment. British Medical Journal 332: 1314.
Lopes P, White J 2006 Heart rate variability: measurement methods and practical implications. In Maud PJ, Foster C (eds) Physiological Assessment of Human Fitness, 2nd edn. Human Kinetics, pp. 39–62.

## Questions for revision

- Draw a diagram illustrating the sequence of electrical activation of different regions of the heart during a normal cardiac cycle. If the sinoatrial node cell action potential was generated at time zero, indicate approximate times at which activation would occur in the bundle of His, the ventricular apices and the atrioventricular margin.

- Draw up a table listing the main characteristics that the heart requires in order to serve its normal function and the mechanisms by which these are achieved.

- Write notes on the functional significance of the slow voltage-gated calcium channels in the heart.

- List typical values for the durations of the P–R interval, the QRS complex and the intervals between the R wave and the beginning and the end of the T wave.

# Chapter 3

# Cardiac output

## CHAPTER CONTENTS

## After reading this chapter, you should:

- understand the factors that determine cardiac output
- know the mechanisms by which cardiac output is increased during exercise
- know the importance of intraventricular turbulence
- be able to assess which methods for non-invasive measurement of cardiac output are most appropriate for use at rest and during exercise.

## FACTORS THAT DETERMINE CARDIAC OUTPUT

In an average-sized subject at rest, the cardiac output of approximately 5 L/min is provided by a stroke volume of around 70 mL pumped at a frequency of around 70 beats/min. Whenever metabolic demand rises there is a need for greater volume delivery of blood around the body. Our capacity to perform whole-body exercise is limited primarily by the upper limit to cardiac output which, in an untrained individual, is around 450% of the value at rest, that is around 22 L/min. The absolute difference between resting and maximal cardiac outputs provides an index of how much metabolic activity can be serviced during exercise and is often termed the *cardiac reserve*.

If you consider the sequence of events reviewed in Chapter 2 you will see that the volume of blood that can be pumped by the heart will be determined by a number of factors including the frequency of pumping, the efficiency of ventricular filling and the efficiency of ventricular emptying.

## Heart rate

The usual resting heart rate of 65–75 beats/min reflects a substantial degree of bradycardic vagal tone, so heart rate can be increased moderately either by reducing that vagal influence or by increasing sympathetic tachycardic drive, or both. Any increase above the intrinsic pacemaker frequency of 100 beats/min, however, relies entirely on sympathetic activation. The sympathetic nerves act through activation of β-adrenoceptors and drugs that antagonize this action (the so-called *β-blockers*) are frequently used in patients for whom exercise is prescribed as a rehabilitative aid after heart attacks. The reduced capacity to produce normal tachycardia is an important factor in determining the absolute intensities of exercise that these individuals are able to undertake and must also be borne in mind if absolute heart rate is being used to quantify their exercise workload (see Chapter 11, p. 131).

With ageing there is a progressive reduction in the capacity of cardiac β-adrenoceptors to respond to sympathetically released catecholamines. In consequence, the absolute maximum to which heart rate can rise during exercise declines with age, being around 200 beats/min at age 20 years, but falling by around 1 beat/min per year. This imposes a progressive limit to cardiac output in older individuals, regardless of their physical fitness.

The standard equation to calculate maximum heart rate ($HR_{max}$) for an adult of a known age is:

$$HR_{max} = 220 - [\text{age in years}]$$

but it is important to bear in mind that this can be applied only to adult subjects. In children, maximum heart rate appears to vary little or not at all with age and remains around a little more than 200 beats/min until approximately 18 years (see Chapter 9, p. 113). In addition, the generalization of $HR_{max}$ falling by 1 beat/min per year has been derived from population studies, and absolute maxima vary by up to 10 beats/min between people of any given age. For this reason, if heart rate is to be used for quantifying workload during exercise then it is preferable to determine each individual's $HR_{max}$ directly.

In obese adults (BMI >30), the relationship between maximal heart rate and age is slightly different and the equation:

$$HR_{max} = 200 - 0.5 [\text{age in years}]$$

appears to be more accurate than the standard one (Miller et al 1993).

# Ventricular filling time

Simple calculation would indicate that a threefold elevation of heart rate should increase cardiac output by the same amount, but it is clear from looking at the pressure–flow relationships during the cardiac cycle (Fig. 3.1) that the situation is not as straightforward as this. As heart rate increases, the interval between successive ventricular contractions decreases so that the absolute time available for refilling falls. With moderate tachycardia this is not a major problem, since most filling occurs during the first 100 ms of diastole when the atrioventricular pressure gradient is greatest. As heart rate increases further, however, filling efficiency falls dramatically. With typical ventricular action potential durations of 300–350 ms it can be calculated that a heart rate of 180 beats/min (1 beat every 330 ms) would actually allow no time for filling at all. Moreover, if there was no diastolic relaxation period then there could be virtually no coronary perfusion to the left ventricle, so myocardial metabolism could not be sustained. Since maximal exercise capacity involves heart rates in young adults of 200 beats/min and cardiac outputs in excess of 20 L/min, this scenario is clearly too simplistic.

The answer is that, in fact, ventricular action potential duration does not remain constant as heart rate increases, because the sympathetically released catecholamines that produce tachycardia also reduce the cycle time of the voltage-gated calcium channels (Fig. 3.2). In consequence, the normal $HR_{max}$ for a 20-year-old of 200 beats/min is associated with an endocardial ventricular action potential plateau phase of about 200 ms rather than the 350 ms seen at rest, allowing around 100 ms for ventricular filling. In consequence, stroke volume falls only slightly even at maximal work capacity.

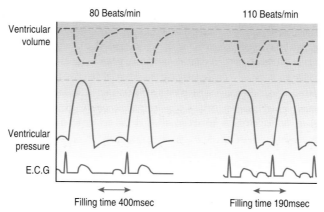

**Figure 3.1** Simulated ventricular pressure and volume curves at 80 and 110 beats/min in a heart with constant ventricular action potential duration. Note that even this moderate increase in heart rate causes a dramatic reduction of ventricular filling time and reduces stroke volume significantly.

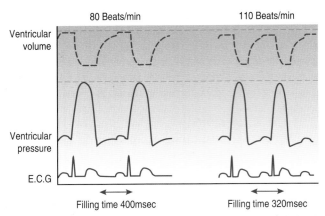

**Figure 3.2** Simulated ventricular pressure and volume curves at 80 and 110 beats/min in a heart with ventricular action potential duration reduced as heart rate increases. Note the improved filling time and stroke volume, compared with Figure 3.1.

## Atrial function

For any finite diastolic period available for ventricular filling, the efficiency of the filling process depends on the pressure gradient between atria and ventricles. This is itself determined by the efficiency of atrial filling, which reflects the pressure gradient from the peripheral veins to the heart. During exercise, two factors facilitate venous return. One is the increased negative pressure inside the thorax during inspiration that results from larger tidal volume. The other is external compression of veins in the moving limbs by muscle contraction (*muscle pumping*) and in the abdomen by abdominal wall muscle activity during expiration. The importance of the leg muscle pump for efficient cardiac filling is illustrated by comparing circulatory responses to arm and leg exercise. During arm exercise, heart rate rises more with given work increments, because the absence of muscle pumping limits stroke volume (see Chapter 7, p. 89).

The atrioventricular pressure gradient is increased directly by increased atrial filling, since this stretches the atrial walls towards their elastic limit so that intra-atrial pressure rises. In addition, activation of atrial β-adrenoceptors by sympathetically released noradrenaline (norepinephrine) and circulating adrenaline (epinephrine) speeds up action potential spread through the atrial syncytium and opens more voltage-gated calcium channels, causing larger amounts of extracellular calcium to enter the atrial cells thereby increasing sarcomere activation (increased *contractility*). These processes both increase active pressure development during atrial contraction.

## Ventricular function

The net consequence of the atrial processes described above is that end-diastolic ventricular volume and pressure rise progressively with exercise until around 60% of maximum work capacity. There are no further changes at workloads higher than this, for three reasons: first, the ongoing reduction in diastolic time limits atrial filling; second, at diastolic volumes above a certain value the ventricular muscle begins to reach its elastic limits and so becomes relatively non-distensible; and third, at these high volumes ventricular expansion becomes restricted also by the stiff pericardial sac that surrounds the heart.

Increased ventricular filling will itself increase stroke volume, due to the Frank-Starling relationship of muscle stretch and active pressure development. In the presence of sympathetic activation, however, systolic pressure generation rises even more, due to the same effects of catecholamines on calcium channel opening as occurs in the atria. The consequences of increased contractility and more rapid contraction of the ventricular syncytium lead to an absolute reduction in end-systolic ventricular volume, so that stroke volume rises with moderate tachycardia even though diastolic filling time is reduced (Fig. 3.3).

## Ventricular afterload

Just as the atrioventricular pressure gradient influences ventricular filling, the pressure gradient between ventricles and arteries must affect the efficiency of ventricular ejection. A higher diastolic arterial pressure must delay equalization of ventricular and arterial pressures during the isovolumetric phase of ventricular contraction, so shortening the proportion of systole during which ejection occurs. In theory, therefore, cardiac output should be elevated most effectively when diastolic blood pressure is minimized. In practice, however, as we shall see in Chapter 7 (p. 85), certain types of exercise are associated

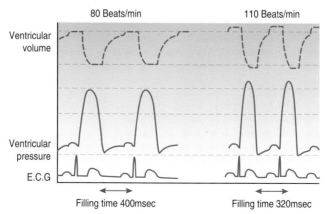

**Figure 3.3** Simulated ventricular pressure and volume curves at 80 and 110 beats/min in a heart with ventricular action potential duration reduced and myocardial contractility increased as heart rate increases. Note that despite the reduced filling time (compare with Fig. 3.2), stroke volume is now higher at the higher heart rate, due to both increased ventricular filling and increased ventricular emptying.

with increased diastolic pressure, so this can be regarded as a further factor in setting the upper effective limit for cardiac performance.

Figure 3.4 shows how the factors discussed above contribute to the exercise response.

## CHARACTERISTICS OF CARDIAC EJECTION

### Turbulent flow

When fluid such as blood is pushed through tubes at low velocities, the particles move parallel to the tube wall and to each other, a state known as laminar flow. Under these conditions, all the energy applied to the fluid is used to move it. At sufficiently high flow velocities, however, the particles begin to interact radially with each other, resulting in swirling movement within the fluid that is termed *turbulence*. Since under these circumstances energy is expended in the inter-particle collisions, turbulent flow is less efficient than laminar flow with respect to the amount of applied force (that is, the pressure gradient) required to move a given volume of fluid through the tube. Turbulent and laminar flow also differ in that the collisions of fluid particles in turbulent flow create a noise, while laminar flow is silent.

With equal volumes of fluid movement per unit time, flow velocity is higher in narrow than wide tubes, so turbulence should be more likely in a narrow tube. Paradoxically, however, turbulence is also facilitated by large tube diameter; so absolute flow velocities that are not high enough to create turbulent flow in narrow tubes may produce turbulence in larger ones. During the cardiac cycle, the absolute velocity of blood flow is highest during the early part of ventricular ejection, when intraventricular pressure is still

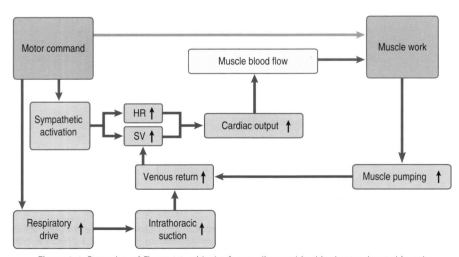

**Figure 3.4** Expansion of Figure 1.1, with the factors discussed in this chapter denoted in red.

rising. Normally, this velocity is slightly less than that required to produce turbulence in tubes the size of the aorta and pulmonary arterial trunk. It does, however, cause turbulence in the larger diameter environment of the ventricle itself. This serves a valuable purpose.

Blood draining back to the right heart from different organs contains varying amounts of secreted hormones, oxygen and carbon dioxide, reflecting the different functions and metabolic rates of the tissues involved. Similarly, blood returning to the left heart from different parts of the lung varies significantly in gas content, reflecting regional variation in the efficiency of ventilation/perfusion matching. These different venous returns are usually not well mixed when they enter the heart, because laminar flow keeps them separate. In consequence, the end-diastolic left ventricular content is far from homogenous in composition and, since arterial flow is also laminar, this creates the potential for different organs to receive blood with different gas tensions and to receive variable amounts of essential hormones. Intraventricular turbulence during the initial phase of systolic ejection ensures homogeneity of the blood delivered to all tissues.

## Heart sounds

The rapid pressure and flow changes in the heart during its pumping action generate noises that can be detected at the surface of the chest wall using a microphone or a stethoscope. These heart sounds constitute what is also known as the *phonocardiogram* and provide important information about the mechanical events that occur during the cardiac cycle. What is termed the first heart sound begins coincidently with the beginning of ventricular contraction and finishes shortly after the beginning of systolic ejection. It involves two sequential events. One corresponds to shutting of the atrioventricular valves as soon as intraventricular pressure begins to rise. The physical closure of the valves does not itself produce noise because they consist of very soft tissue, but the sudden cessation of blood movement causes vibration of the ventricular walls. This sound is followed without pause by a longer-lasting component due to the fast turbulent phase of systolic ejection. What is termed the second heart sound corresponds to the end of systole, when the rapid fall in intraventricular pressure reverses the pressure gradient between arteries and ventricles and the semi-lunar valves shut. These valves consist of relatively stiff tissue and so, unlike the situation with the atrioventricular valves and the first heart sound, the noise created directly reflects their shutting.

Because the heart sounds have a predictable relationship to mechanical events, they can be used to time the cardiac cycle (Fig. 3.5). Thus, the period between the beginning of the first and second sounds must define the period during which the ventricles are contracting. More important, since the isovolumetric phase of systole is short and varies only relatively little over a wide range of afterloads, the period between first and second sounds approximates the duration of ejection. Although the interval between R and T waves

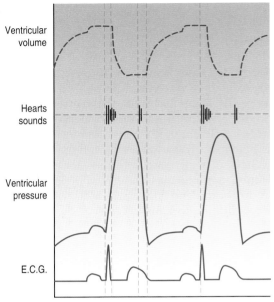

Ventricular volume

Hearts sounds

Ventricular pressure

E.C.G.

**Figure 3.5** Timing of the first and second heart sounds relative to pressure and flow changes during the cardiac cycle. Note that the first sound occurs during both isovolumetric contraction and the initial phase of ventricular ejection, while the second sound is much shorter and defines the cessation of ejection.

in the ECG also gives some information on this, timing of the end of ejection from the ECG is uncertain because of the long timecourse of the T wave.

The events that dictate whether flow is laminar or turbulent, together with the basis for the heart sounds, mean that altered heart sounds can be used to detect a variety of defects of cardiac function. For instance, failure of the atrioventricular valves to close fully (*valvular incompetence*) would lead to retrograde leakage at high pressure during ventricular contraction. This produces turbulent noise during systolic ejection and so prolongs the first sound. Similarly, incompetence of the semi-lunar valves causes turbulent backflow at the end of systole and so prolongs the second sound. Finally, if the semi-lunar valves do not open fully (*valvular stenosis*) then the velocity of blood flow into the central arteries will be increased and create turbulent noise that may last through the entire ejection period.

## PRACTICAL APPROACHES TO MEASUREMENT OF CARDIAC OUTPUT

For satisfactory use in normal healthy subjects, it is important that the techniques used to measure cardiovascular parameters are non-invasive wherever possible. This minimizes potential for adverse events, is more comfortable for subjects and is more likely to encourage participation. A variety of non-invasive approaches is available for estimation of cardiac output. The choice between these depends on the accuracy required, the technologies that are to hand and the experimental environment. The following section summarizes the principles underlying those methods that are in common use and indicates their advantages and limitations.

## Extrapolation from oxygen consumption

Some years ago (Astrand et al 1964) it was shown that with workloads below the lactate threshold cardiac output can be estimated from oxygen consumption according to the following equations, where both cardiac output and oxygen consumption are expressed in L/min:

$$\text{males : cardiac output} = 6.55 + 4.35 \, [O_2 \text{ consumption}]$$
$$\text{females : cardiac output} = 3.66 + 6.81 \, [O_2 \text{ consumption}]$$

Although these equations were based on careful experimentation, they may not give accurate values for cardiac output under some circumstances and more direct techniques of measurement are usually preferable. Even then, as will be seen below, the available methods all have certain limitations if they are to be applied to an exercising subject.

## Application of the Fick principle to carbon–dioxide production

Carbon dioxide is produced continually by the peripheral tissues and cleared into the alveolar air. If one measures whole-body production by collecting expired air and simultaneously measures the difference in carbon-dioxide concentration across the pulmonary circulation, then these figures can be used to calculate the volume of blood that was necessary to deliver the expired carbon dioxide. Take for example the following typical values:

$$\text{pulmonary arterial } [CO_2] - 52 \text{ mL/100 mL blood}$$
$$\text{pulmonary venous } [CO_2] - 48 \text{ mL/100 mL blood}$$
$$\text{whole-body } CO_2 \text{ production} - 200 \text{mL/min}$$

From the difference between pulmonary arterial and pulmonary venous contents, each 100 mL blood loses 4 mL $CO_2$ as it passes through the lung. If total $CO_2$ production is 200 mL/min then pulmonary blood flow (that is, cardiac output) over the same time must be:

$$(200/4)100 \text{ mL} = 50.100 \text{ mL} = 5000 \text{ mL}$$

that is, cardiac output is 5 L/min.

In practice, the rapid equilibration of $CO_2$ between blood and alveolar air means that we do not need to measure blood concentrations of $CO_2$ directly in order to make reasonably accurate estimates of cardiac output, provided that pulmonary function is normal and the subject is at a steady state for $CO_2$ production. The end-expiratory $CO_2$ concentration can be regarded as in equilibrium with that leaving the lung in the pulmonary venous blood ($PaCO_2$) and this can be calculated as:

$$PaCO_2 = 5.5 + 0.90 \text{ [end-exp } CO_2] - 0.0021 \text{ [tidal volume] (Myers 1996)}$$

and then converted to arterial $CO_2$ content by reference to a $CO_2$ dissociation table. The assumption that complete equilibrium is achieved between air and plasma has to be recognized as a potential source of error, because the steep slope of the $CO_2$ dissociation curve means that significant changes in $CO_2$ content could occur with only minor shifts in alveolar $PCO_2$.

Pulmonary arterial $CO_2$ concentration ($P_vCO_2$) is approximately 6 mmHg higher than $PaCO_2$, under almost all circumstances in normal individuals, regardless of whether they are at rest or exercising. Accurate measurement of $PvCO_2$, however, requires a rebreathing technique. The subject breathes into a bag that contains oxygen plus a concentration of around 10% $CO_2$, which is significantly higher than $PvCO_2$. This reversal of the normal concentration gradient causes $CO_2$ to diffuse into the bloodstream until, after a few breaths, alveolar and plasma concentrations equilibrate and the $PCO_2$ remaining in the bag is identical to $P_vCO_2$.

With continuous gas analysis using a metabolic cart and approximation of $P_vCO_2$ this technique allows cardiac output determination on a breath-to-breath basis. The rebreathing procedure, however, requires around 5 or 6 breaths, so accurate measurements can be made only around once per minute. Clearly it is not technically feasible to measure true beat-to-beat output (stroke volume).

## Nitrous oxide rebreathing

This is another method that employs the Fick principle, but which measures pulmonary exchange of a foreign gas as a marker rather than that of endogenous $CO_2$. The subject breathes from a bag of oxygen containing known concentrations of a soluble inert gas (usually nitrous oxide) and of an insoluble gas such as sulphur hexafluoride. The rate of decrease in nitrous oxide concentration in the bag must be proportional to the rate at which it is taken up by the pulmonary bloodstream, and computer algorithms allow the volume flow involved to be calculated. In healthy lungs, the only other factor that could affect gas uptake is a change in pulmonary exchange area caused by altered depth of ventilation. This is adjusted for by monitoring any change in the concentration of the insoluble marker. The inert gas technique avoids the approximations that are inherent with methods that use $CO_2$ and the literature suggests that this method provides closely similar values of cardiac output to those obtained using invasive techniques in the same subjects. For the purposes of the exercise physiologist, its main limitation is that all the absorbed nitrous oxide has to be expired again before a second measurement can be made. In practice this means that successive measurements can be obtained only once every several minutes, which can limit the accuracy of tracking cardiac output during graded exercise.

## Thoracic conductance and impedance

If the resting electrical resistance of the thorax is measured along the rostro-caudal axis, a decreased resistance can be detected during the rostral movement of blood into the aortic arch that is associated with cardiac ejection. The magnitude of this change is proportional to the volume of blood involved and is, therefore, an index of stroke volume. Resistance measurement is by means of adhesive skin electrodes positioned above and below the rostro-caudal limits of the heart and stroke volume is calculated using an algorithm that incorporates the resistivity of blood and the period of ejection as measured from the ECG or a phonocardiogram.

These techniques have been calibrated against invasive methods for assessment of cardiac output. They appear acceptably accurate and are able to provide beat-to-beat measurement of cardiac output at rest and during light to moderate whole-body stationery exercise. With intense exercise, however, movement artefacts preclude readable records and, with prolonged exercise or exposure to heat, sweat-induced loss of electrode adhesion becomes a problem.

## Imaging

Like the impedance and conductance techniques, Doppler echocardiography provides beat-to-beat information on stroke volume. It involves simultaneous determination of aortic arch diameter and the velocity of blood flow through this vessel, by means of a detector placed manually on the thoracic wall. The technique is reliable for assessing cardiac output at rest, but it relies on very accurate and stable positioning of the imaging detector on the skin. Therefore, although it could be employed during exercise that involves only lower body movements it is not useful in any circumstances where the subject is ambulatory.

## Key points

Substantial increases in cardiac output over resting values can be achieved only if tachycardia is accompanied by shortened ejection time.

The maximal achievable heart rate is a useful marker of maximal exercise capacity and can be approximated in adults by simple calculations if age is known.

The heart sounds provide markers of ejection period and can be used to check the normality of cardiac valvular function.

A number of non-invasive methods exist for measurement of cardiac output, but all have limitations of use during exercise and most are able to provide intermittent rather than beat-to-beat data.

## References

Astrand P, Cuddy PTE, Saltin B, Stenberg J 1964 Cardiac output during submaximal and maximal work. Journal of Applied Physiology 19: 268–274.
Miller WC, Wallace JP, Eggert KE 1993 Predicting max HR and the HR-$VO_2$ relationship for exercise prescription in obesity. Medicine and Science of Sports and Exercise 25: 1077–1081.

## Further reading

Hayes B 1997 Doppler ultrasound monitoring, including echocardiography. In: Non-Invasive Cardiovascular Monitoring. BMJ Publishing, London, Chapter 13.
Hayes B 1997 Electrical impedance monitoring. In: Non-Invasive Cardiovascular Monitoring. BMJ Publishing, London, Chapter 14.
Myers JN 1996 Essentials of Cardiopulmonary Exercise Testing. Human Kinetics, Champaign, IL.
Peyton PJ, Thompson B 2004 Agreement of an inert gas rebreathing device with thermodilution and the direct oxygen Fick method in measurement of pulmonary blood flow. Journal of Clinical Monitoring 18: 373–378.

**Questions for revision**

- As heart rate increases, the time for ventricular filling must decrease. How is it, then, that cardiac output rises as heart rate rises?

- A typical 30-year-old man has a maximal heart rate of about 190 beats/min and a resting heart rate of 70 beats/min. This means that increasing his heart rate to its maximum can be calculated to increase his cardiac output by a factor of 190/70 or 2.7-fold. However, during maximal exercise cardiac output rises typically by four-fold. How is this achieved?

- What are the relative advantages and limitations of the various methods by which cardiac output can be measured non-invasively in human subjects?

# Chapter **4**

# Blood-pressure generation

## CHAPTER CONTENTS

### After reading this chapter, you should:

- **understand the factors that determine arterial blood pressure**
- **be able to predict how systolic, diastolic and pulse pressures will be changed by altered cardiac performance and peripheral resistance**
- **be able to assess which methods for measurement of blood pressure are most appropriate at rest and during exercise**

Together with heart rate, pulsatile blood pressure is the most readily accessible measure of cardiovascular performance in humans. Blood pressure rises with sympathetic activation and this pressor response plays a vital role in optimizing blood flow to muscle and other vital organs during exercise. It is, therefore, important to spend a little time considering the factors that determine the limits of pressure pulsation and how these will be affected by increased sympathetic drive. The changes in blood pressure that occur during exercise will be examined in more detail in Chapter 7.

## FACTORS AFFECTING BLOOD PRESSURE

### Limits to blood pressure

#### Systolic pressure

The extent to which blood pressure rises during systolic ejection reflects how much the energy of ejection is able to compress the arterial contents downstream of the left ventricle. The size of the stroke volume is, therefore, one obvious factor that will influence the level of systolic blood pressure (SBP). Anything that reduces stroke volume will reduce SBP (Fig. 4.1A,B). In normal individuals, the most usual situations in which this occurs is when cardiac filling falls because of an increase in heart rate or reduced venous return, typically during postural change.

The linkage of stroke volume to SBP means that this pressure can in normal individuals be used to assess cardiac workload, most commonly by calculating the product of heart rate and SBP, termed the *rate–pressure product*. By contrast, in hearts where the atrioventricular valves do not seal fully so that there is back-flow of a proportion of the stroke volume or the semilunar valves do not open fully so that ejection of blood is delayed, then stroke volume and SBP are reduced but intraventricular pressure is increased. Under these circumstances, SBP can no longer be used as an index of cardiac work; in fact, there is likely to be an inverse relationship between the two.

Under most circumstances, not all of the energy developed by the myocardium during ejection is translated into pressure, because the proximal part of the aorta is distensible (*compliant*) rather than being a rigid tube and a proportion of ejection energy is, therefore, stored as potential energy as the aortic wall is stretched. The functional value of this is that once ejection is complete, aortic elastic recoil will continue to exert intravascular pressure and provide a means of converting the purely pulsatile cardiac ejection into continuous flow through the peripheral circulation.

Generalised sympathetic nervous system activation elevates SBP, due to a variety of factors. First, increased cardiac muscle contractility reduces

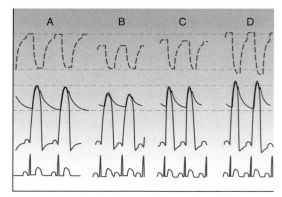

**Figure 4.1** Effects on pulsatile aortic blood pressure (red) of varying left ventricular function. (A) Typical normal relationship between blood pressure and (from top downwards) ventricular volume, ventricular pressure and ECG. In (B), heart rate has increased without changed ventricular mechanical function; this reduces SBP due to reduced ventricular filling. In (C), the same heart rate increase is accompanied by shortening of the ventricular action potential, improving ventricular filling and returning SBP towards the control value. (D) The full physiological response to tachycardia, with action potential shortening, increased myocardial contractility and aortic stiffening: now, SBP is elevated above control, reflecting the increased stroke volume. Note that while tachycardia elevates DBP because of the reduced time for arterial run-off, this effect remains virtually the same regardless of stroke volume.

end-systolic ventricular volume and increases stroke volume. Second, an increased action potential conduction velocity through the ventricular myocardium leads to faster compression of the contents and, therefore, to a higher velocity of ejection. In addition, the smooth muscle in the proximal aorta receives a sympathetic innervation and contraction of these muscle cells reduces aortic compliance. This stiffening allows all of the energy of ejection to be used in pressure generation. Finally, sympathetic vasoconstrictor drive to veins stiffens these and mobilizes blood normally stored in the venous reservoir back into active circulation, aiding cardiac filling and further increasing stroke volume. The additive effects of these factors are illustrated in Figures 4.1C and D.

### Diastolic pressure

As diastolic blood pressure (DBP) represents the lowest value to which pressure falls in the arteries before the next systolic ejection, it must be influenced by the period over which the pressure can fall, so heart rate itself is also a major determinant of DBP, with tachycardia predictably causing a pressure rise (Fig. 4.1). Heart rate changes will also affect SBP if pulse pressure remains constant but, in practice, the consequences of heart rate alteration for ventricular filling time and, therefore, for stroke volume tends to minimize SBP changes.

The second main influence on DBP is the rate at which intra-arterial pressure falls after systolic ejection ceases; that is, how fast the pressurized blood flows out through the resistance of the peripheral blood vessels. Thus, the *total peripheral resistance* is a major determinant of DBP and changes in DBP can in many situations be used as an index of peripheral resistance changes. While all vascular beds and all segments of the vasculature contribute to the overall resistance of the system, most of the peripheral resistance occurs in the largest regional vascular beds, those supplying the digestive tract and associated tissues (the *splanchnic* circulation), the skeletal muscles, the skin and the kidneys, and almost all is localized to the arteriolar segment of the vasculature. In Chapter 5 (p. 50) we will see why the arterioles produce so much more resistance to flow than do other parts of the vascular tree.

Figure 4.2 adds the effects of sympathetic activation on cardiac generation of blood pressure to our flow chart of the exercise response.

## Mean versus phasic arterial pressure

As indicated above, the phasic limits of blood pressure can provide valuable information on the behaviour of specific components of the circulatory system. The pulsatile nature of pressure in large arteries is, however, irrelevant to perfusion of the peripheral tissues, since virtually all pulsatility is damped out by the time blood enters the capillaries. Also, calculation of parameters such as peripheral resistance requires an averaged value for

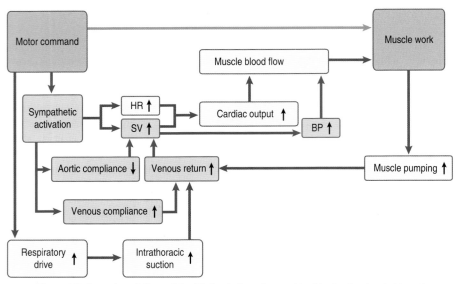

**Figure 4.2** Expansion of Figure 3.4, with the factors discussed in this chapter denoted in red.

pressure. The concept of *mean arterial pressure* is, therefore, essential to quantitative evaluation of circulatory function.

### Does mean blood pressure change with heart rate?

As mean pressure represents the average value throughout the cardiac cycle and the shape of the pulse wave means that the pressure is closer to DBP than to SBP for much of the cycle, the mean cannot simply be taken as half way between the two limits. For practical purposes it is assumed to lie approximately one-third (actually $1/e$) of the way up the pressure waveform and so can be calculated as:

$$\text{mean BP} = \frac{\text{DBP} + 1}{3\text{PP}}$$

or

$$\text{mean BP} = \frac{(\text{SBP} + 2\text{DBP})}{3}$$

With increasing heart rate, the shape of the BP wave changes so that the flatter late diastolic portion disappears and the waveform becomes more triangular. There is some experimental evidence suggesting that under these circumstances mean BP may be better approximated by DBP + 2/5PP (Robinson et al 1988).

## Central and peripheral arterial pressures

The concept of arterial pressure generation from cardiac ejection and the factors determining systolic and diastolic limits as discussed above relate specifically to pressure just outside the semilunar valves. In the systemic circulation, however, additional factors become significant in pressure determination the further one moves away from the heart down the system of distributing arteries, with the result that absolute values recorded from, for example, arteries in the arm or leg, are no longer a precise reflection of the pressures in the aortic arch.

A finite resistance to flow is imposed by the vessel walls, so that mean BP falls progressively along the arterial tree. If this were not the case, there would be no pressure gradient and no flow could occur. For the same reason, DBP falls to a similar extent. Nonetheless, this longitudinal resistance to flow is quite small in large arteries so that the mean BP and DBP fall by only around 5 mmHg between the aortic arch and the brachial artery at the elbow.

By contrast, SBP in the brachial and other peripheral conducting arteries may be up to 10–15 mmHg higher than in the aortic arch. This change is due in part to reflection of pressure when the descending pressure wave meets the much higher resistance of the microcirculation. As well, the more peripheral arteries lack the high compliance of the thoracic aorta, so the energy of cardiac contraction is no longer partially dissipated in volume changes of the vessels.

## MEASUREMENT OF ARTERIAL PRESSURE

### Palpation

The sudden rise in intra-arterial pressure associated with systole can be detected with the fingertips in a number of arteries that lie just below the skin surface. The most commonly used site is the radial artery at the wrist. If an occlusive cuff is inflated around the arm, the pulsation disappears once the cuff is inflated above SBP and reappears during deflation when cuff pressure falls below SBP. This is a rapid method for determining SBP. It can provide no information on DBP and so cannot be used for calculation of mean BP.

### Auscultation

Auscultation (from the Latin *ausculatatus* = to listen to) is the traditional method by which blood pressure is detected using a stethoscope or a microphone applied to the skin over an artery, distal to an occlusive cuff. While it is routine to apply the cuff to the upper arm and the detector to the brachial artery at the elbow, this technique can also be used to measure pressure in the patellar artery at the knee.

The technique relies on the luminal diameter of an artery being narrowed along the section underneath an inflated occlusive cuff and that this diameter suddenly increases at the downstream edge of the cuff. Flow velocity is increased through the narrowed section of the vessel. The combination of this increased velocity and the larger diameter vessel just downstream of the cuff transforms the flow profile to a turbulent one just in this region. At occlusive pressures above SBP there is of course no forward flow and so no turbulence. At pressures below SBP, however, intra-arterial pressure exceeds the cuff pressure for a portion of each cardiac cycle, producing periods of noisy turbulent flow separated by silence. These noises are known as *Korotkow sounds*.

During inspiration, the increased cardiac filling and consequent increased stroke volume associated with negative intrathoracic pressure causes a rise in SBP. In younger individuals, this is reinforced by the tachycardic phase of sinus arrhythmia. Appreciable respiratory fluctuations in SBP are seen even during quiet respiration, and are more pronounced at low respiratory frequencies because the longer period of low intrathoracic pressure allows greater cardiac filling (Fig. 4.3). In order to measure SBP accurately, it is obviously important that the cuff is inflated to a pressure that is above the highest SBP value. The standard recommendation is for inflation to a value around 20 mmHg higher than that at which the palpated radial pulse disappears, but this advice does not take account of the respiratory phase at which the pulse is detected. For accurate results, it is a sensible precaution to measure several palpated SBP values over a complete respiratory cycle and then to use an inflation pressure for auscultation around 20 mmHg above the maximum recorded.

During deflation of the cuff, blood flow becomes almost continuous once the occlusive pressure falls to within a few mmHg of DBP, because of the flattened base of the pulse wave. This transition from intermittent to near-continuous flow is detected through the stethoscope as a change in the character of the Korotkow sounds from discrete tapping to a more blurred and somewhat softer noise, a change known as 'muffling', or Korotkow phase IV. Once cuff pressure falls below a value approximating DBP, the amount of vessel distortion is insufficient to cause turbulence in the presence of absolute blood flow velocities typical of normal resting cardiac output. Therefore, the cuff pressure at which Korotkow sounds disappear (Korotkow phase V) can be used as an approximation of DBP. This is convenient because the presence or absence of a sound is usually easier to assess than whether the character of the sound has changed, especially when there is a high level of background noise.

However, it is essential for the experimental scientist to remember that the association of Korotkow phase V with DBP is coincidental and based entirely on the absolute velocity of blood flow. If velocity increases because cardiac output is elevated (for example by exercise or pregnancy), or because the occluded artery is small in diameter (as occurs in children), then

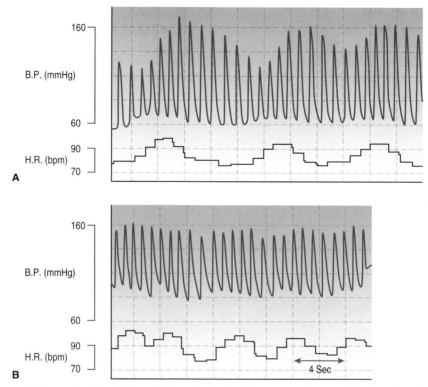

**Figure 4.3** Fluctuations in SBP during quiet breathing in a healthy, 24-year-old woman. The phase of inspiration can be identified by the progressive tachycardia. (A) With slow respiration at 7 breaths/min, the increased cardiac filling and stroke volume associated with inspiration increases SBP by up to 50 mmHg. (B) At a respiratory frequency of 15 breaths/min in the same subject, the duration of negative intrathoracic pressure is shortened and the amplitude of SBP fluctuation is reduced correspondingly.

less compression of the artery will be sufficient to cause turbulence. Under these circumstances, Korotkow sounds may persist until cuff pressure is as much as 20–30 mmHg below DBP. By contrast, the cuff pressure at which muffling occurs has a constant and close relationship to DBP. For this reason, muffling and not disappearance of sounds must be used as the auscultatory criterion for DBP during exercise if serious errors are to be avoided. A stethoscope is essential in such circumstances: microphones are able to reliably recognize only the presence or absence of sounds.

Robinson et al (1988) proposed on the basis of comparisons of auscultatory and inter-arterial BP values that the standard formula DBP + 1/3PP does not provide accurate calculation of mean BP when auscultatory readings are used during heavy exercise; it was suggested that DBP + 1/2PP gave a closer approximation of true (that is, intra-arterial) mean pressure. However, the intra-arterial values in that study were significantly higher than those from auscultation and appeared likely to be an overestimate of the true pressure because of the cannula placement (see Intra-arterial catheters, below).

If this probable error is discounted then there seems no good reason to assume that the standard formula is not accurate even at high work intensities.

A number of alternative methods for BP measurement are available and in some situations provide advantages over the auscultatory technique. These are summarized below. However, auscultation is the most generally appropriate for obtaining accurate values during whole-body exercise and, therefore, it is important that every exercise physiologist is expert in its use.

## HANDY HINTS

The sphygmomanometer cuff used for auscultation is pressurized by pumping a hand-held rubber bulb and deflated by opening a needle valve. Practice, so that you can pump the bulb and regulate the valve using one hand only, since you will need your other hand for holding the stethoscope. When inflating the cuff, fully squash the bulb every time you squeeze it so that the pressure rises as fast as possible. Slow pressure rises obstruct venous return before the arterial flow is cut off, which causes tissue swelling in the forearm and makes it more difficult to hear the Korotkow sounds. It is also essential not to leave the cuff inflated for longer than necessary, as this becomes uncomfortable so the subject is, therefore, no longer relaxed and, thus, blood pressure may rise. To obtain accurate pressure readings, you need during cuff deflation to be able to control the rate of pressure fall between around 2 mmHg/s and 5 mmHg/s.

To hear the Korotkow sounds well, the stethoscope head must be sealed against the skin, but not pressed so firmly that it compresses the artery. If you are listening in the antecubital fossa at the elbow, good apposition without excessive pressure is most easily achieved by cupping your hand round the arm with your thumb pressing very lightly on the back of the stethoscope head and your fingers supporting the elbow. Alternatively, place the stethoscope on the inner surface of the upper arm just proximal to the medial epicondyle and once again use your thumb to hold it gently against the skin while you cup your fingers around the elbow. Since absolute intra-arterial pressure is affected by gravity, the stethoscope head should be kept at about the same vertical level as the heart. However, small differences between heart and cuff level are not really worth worrying about. A vertical difference of 1 cm will change pressure by less than 1 mmHg.

In a few individuals the Korotkow sounds disappear and then reappear in the middle of the pulse pressure range. The silent range of pressures is known as the 'auscultatory gap' (Korotkow phases II–III). In these individuals, the pressure at which sounds reappear might be mistaken for SBP, or the pressure at which they disappear might be mistaken for DBP. It is, therefore, a sensible precaution to always check the cuff pressure at which the palpated radial pulse disappears and reappears, before starting ausculta-tory measurement.

## Oscillometry

This technique is used in the portable blood pressure monitoring kits com-monly available from pharmacies and medical suppliers and in routine hospital units such as the Dinamap™. The occlusive cuff is usually inflated automatically to a preset value and deflates at a preset rate. The absolute pressure inside the cuff is monitored at a high frequency and an algorithm is used to determine which part of the pressure wave corresponds to particular pressure values.

The oscillometric technique has several potential advantages over ausculta-tion. For one thing, the underlying theory obviates the potential problems of detecting and interpreting Korotkow sounds. As well, observer error is removed. Extensive studies of the pressure values recorded using ausculta-tion by even highly trained personnel show that a surprisingly high number of people routinely round numbers up or down, sometimes to the nearest 10 mmHg. The automatic digital display provided by oscillometry avoids this potentially serious source of error. However, since they rely on small variations in cuff pressure for their operation, oscillometric devices are extremely sensitive to movement of the cuff relative to the skin. This means that they cannot be used unless the arm is completely stationary, precluding their use during whole-body exercise.

A further problematic characteristic is the fact that the automated inflation–deflation cycle cannot be overridden easily. If SBP is above the preset inflation ceiling then the cuff immediately deflates without taking a measurement. In experimental circumstances where SBP varies from moment to moment, for example in subjects with pronounced sinus arrhythmia or during laboratory stress tests, this may result in unacceptable loss of data. Alternatively, the inflation ceiling can be preset to a very high value. However, this prolongs the inflation time and is found by some subjects to be uncomfortable, leading to stress-induced hypertension.

## Applanation tonometry

This technique employs high-frequency application of inwardly directed pressure over an artery, so as to continually exactly balance the intravascular pressure. The pressurizing and sensing devices are located together in a housing that is strapped on the skin, overlying either the radial artery at the wrist or a digital artery on a finger. As no process of cuff inflation or deflation is needed, a continuous beat-to-beat record of BP is obtained. This makes the technique an attractive one when SBP varies from moment to moment and for situations in which rapid changes in BP must be tracked.

For example, a Valsalva manoeuvre (see Chapter 10, p. 120) lasts typically for only around 12 s. Over this time there are several significant changes in BP due to different mechanisms, all of which must be measured in order to assess the physiological response. None of these pressure changes could be detected by auscultation or oscillometry because the cuff inflation–deflation cycle takes in excess of 20 s.

Despite this advantage, applanation tonometry has its own limitations. One is that the positioning of the detecting head is critical, so the wrist or finger must be kept absolutely still. In the case of wrist devices, this makes it very difficult to maintain BP measurements during even light exercise. With finger devices, exercise can be performed as long as one hand can be kept motionless, but this obviously restricts both the type and the intensity of exercise undertaken. The finger presents a further problem with anything but short experiments. As the fingers are a major site for thermoregulatory heat exchange, the digital arteries are usually relatively vasoconstricted, which causes a significant fall in pressure from that in the larger, more central arteries. To obviate this error, devices that record from digital arteries include a heating element that ensures local vasodilatation. However, the effect of this can be painful when a finger is exposed for longer than around 30 min. So during prolonged study sessions it is necessary to periodically change fingers, resulting in inevitable gaps in the pressure record.

## Intra-arterial catheters

Of all the above techniques, auscultation is the only one that can give reliable information during intense whole-body exercise. Even then, it has to be accepted that readings are possible only about every 60 s because of the need for slow cuff deflation in order to obtain accurate values. If more frequent readings are necessary, or when blood pressure must be monitored remotely (for instance from swimming subject), then the only alternative is to use direct intra-arterial cannulation. This is not a course to be taken lightly. The procedure requires medical expertise and sterile conditions, it involves some subject discomfort and there is always a small but finite risk of injury. Nonetheless, intra-arterial recording is routine in a number of exercise physiology facilities, most of which are attached to hospitals. Some information on the methodology used can be found in Wasserman et al (2004).

To interpret intra-arterial BP measurements accurately, it is important to know the position of the catheter tip and the direction in which this faces. The catheter is usually inserted retrogradely into the radial artery in the forearm or the femoral artery in the groin and, because of the rise in SBP with increasing distance away from the heart (see Central and peripheral pressures, p. 35), the absolute pressures recorded will depend on how far the cannula tip is advanced towards the central aorta. In addition, most catheters are open-tipped tubes, so when they are inserted retrogradely into an artery the open tip faces upstream. Under these circumstances, the pressure recorded is greater than the true intravascular hydrostatic pressure, because of the kinetic energy of blood flow pushing on the catheter lumen. The kinetic component is determined primarily by the velocity of blood flow and can be calculated as:

$$P_{kinetic} = 1/2.density.velocity^2$$

As flow velocity is greatest during the ejection phase of the cardiac cycle, $P_{kinetic}$ affects SBP more than DBP. At a normal resting cardiac output, it adds around 4–8 mmHg to SBP, but the quadratic relationship to flow velocity means that the contribution rises rapidly as cardiac output rises. If, for example, $P_{kinetic}$ added an additional 5 mmHg to SBP at rest, then a three-fold rise in cardiac output should increase the kinetic contribution by $3^2$ or ninefold, to 45 mmHg. This would introduce a serious source of error if intra-arterial values were compared quantitatively with those obtained by non-invasive techniques in the same subject.

When an end-opening catheter faces downstream, then the true intra-arterial pressure is underestimated by the $P_{kinetic}$ value. This is not a problem with systemic BP measurement but can be important when measuring pulmonary BP, since the catheters for this purpose are inserted through a central vein and passed on through the right heart (see Chapter 8, p. 101). The only way in which the kinetic artefact can be obviated is to use a catheter that has its opening at right angles to the direction of blood flow.

## Case history

A 32-year-old woman athlete (Rita V.) had continued to exercise non-competitively throughout her pregnancy, without any ill effects. During the eighth month of pregnancy, however, she suddenly began to feel dizzy during cycle ergometry at around 60% $\dot{V}O_{2max}$. Some time ago, Rita had decided to monitor her blood pressure daily. She chose a home blood–pressure kit that detected Korotkow sounds with an in-built microphone rather than an oscillometric device, because she wanted to be able to use it during exercise. During her most recent bout of dizziness she recorded her blood pressure as 136/16 mHg. At rest, prior to the exercise, she had recorded values of 126/70 mmHg. Rita was understandably concerned that she could be suffering from inadequate circulation and that her baby may be in danger if she continued to exercise.

## Discussion

This is a nice example of technology getting in the way of biological reality! Home blood-pressure-measuring devices that rely on auscultatory detection of Korotkow sounds have to include an in-built microphone because it would be too difficult to market them with a separate stethoscope. However, anything but the most sophisticated microphone cannot distinguish between different qualities of sound and recognizes only whether the sound is present or absent. By definition, therefore, these devices are constrained to using Korotkow phase V as the index of DBP.

In normal people with normal resting cardiac outputs, there is no significant difference in DBP detected by Korotkow phase IV or phase V. If, on the other hand, the velocity of blood flow through the radial artery is increased substantially above normal resting values, then arterial turbulence may occur with even quite small degrees of arterial compression associated with cuff pressures that may be significantly below DBP. In Rita's case, the velocity of blood flow during moderate exercise alone was not sufficient to cause a large artefactual fall in detected DBP. However, pregnancy itself is associated with a progressive rise in cardiac output, reflecting the progressive increase in fetoplacental blood flow. At eight months of pregnancy, resting cardiac output would be around 1.5 L/min higher than in the non-pregnant state. Superimposition of this effect on arterial flow velocity on the effect of exercise was sufficient to cause turbulent flow even when the artery was minimally compressed.

## MEASUREMENT OF TOTAL PERIPHERAL RESISTANCE

Since the peripheral resistance imposed by the arterial system is an essential regulatory contributor to blood pressure and to cardiac work, measurement of the *total peripheral resistance* (TPR) is often important for interpretation of experiments in which cardiovascular function has been manipulated. Simple qualitative information on changes in TPR can be obtained from changes in DBP since, in the absence of heart rate changes, TPR is the primary factor affecting DBP. Quantitative calculation of TPR requires measurement of both mean blood pressure and cardiac output:

$$TPR = \frac{BP}{CO}$$

so the advantages and limitations of techniques for determining each of these parameters have to be considered for any particular experimental situation. The unit for TPR as derived from this formula can be either (mmHg/mL)/min or (mmHg/L)/min, depending on whether cardiac output is expressed in L/min or mL/min and, rather confusingly, both are usually referred to simply as *peripheral resistance units (PRUs)* rather than citing the individual parameters involved. To avoid confusion, it is important to bear this in mind and be aware that PRUs derived using mL/min will give TPR values of the order of 0.02–0.05 while those derived using L/min give values around 20–50.

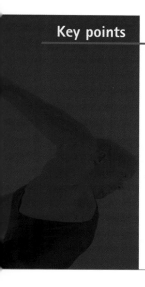

## Key points

Systolic arterial pressure is selectively affected by stroke volume and aortic compliance, while diastolic pressure is selectively affected by heart rate and peripheral resistance.

Although mean intravascular pressure must fall along the length of the arterial system, pulse pressure rises between the aortic arch and the large peripheral arteries.

The traditional auscultatory technique is the only reliable non-invasive method for blood pressure measurement during intense whole-body exercise.

If beat-to-beat pressure measurement is required, then either invasive arterial cannulation must be carried out or exercise intensity must be low enough to not interfere with non-invasive techniques.

## References

Robinson TR, Sue DY, Huszczuk A, Weiler-Ravell D, Hansen JE 1988 Intra-arterial and cuff blood pressure responses during incremental cycle ergometry. Medicine and Science in Sports and Exercise 20: 142–149.

Wasserman K, Hansen JE, Sue DY, Casaburi R, Whipp BJ 1999 Principles of exercise testing and interpretation. Lippincott Williams & Wilkins, Philadelphia, pp. 125–126.

## Further reading

Hayes B 1997 Non-invasive blood pressure (NIBP) monitoring. In: Non-Invasive Cardiovascular Monitoring. BMJ Publishing, London; Chapter 4.

### Questions for revision

- List the factors that affect the absolute values of (i) systolic and (ii) diastolic blood pressures.

- Discuss the effect on blood pressure of increased sympathetic drive to the heart.

- What is the basis for Korotkow sounds and how are these employed in auscultatory measurement of blood pressure?

- List the advantages and limitations of the different non-invasive methods for measuring blood pressure.

# Chapter 5

# Vascular system

## CHAPTER CONTENTS

## After reading this chapter, you should:

- understand the factors that determine peripheral vascular resistance
- appreciate the differences between flow in rigid and distensible vessels
- know the effects of Laplace's law on the circulation
- know the usual techniques for assessment of arterial distensibility and blood flows to skin and muscle
- be able to describe the ways in which structural specialization of vessels can be important in optimizing the transfer functions of the circulation

The volume flow of blood around the circulation per unit time ($\dot{Q}$) can be expressed in terms of the pressure gradient ($\Delta P$) and the absolute resistance to flow of the vasculature (R):

$$\dot{Q} = \frac{\Delta P}{R}$$

Intravascular pressure at the downstream end of the vascular circuit where it drains into the heart is virtually the same as atmospheric pressure and can be regarded as 0 mmHg. The value of $\Delta P$, therefore, depends primarily on the value of arterial blood pressure. In the last chapter we looked at the aspects of cardiac function that affect this and reviewed briefly the involvement of the peripheral vasculature. We need now to examine in more detail the properties of blood vessels and how these contribute to resistance to flow.

## PHYSICAL FACTORS AFFECTING PERIPHERAL RESISTANCE

### Vessel length

The pressure of fluid flowing through a tube falls progressively along the tube, due to friction between the fluid and the tube wall. Thus, vessels of different lengths must contribute differently to overall peripheral resistance, with short vascular beds such as that of the stomach having less resistance (and correspondingly faster circulation times) than those of the limbs.

Even though some vessels travel in the walls of organs that change size dramatically, such as the bladder, stretching of these organs does not alter the length of the vessels. When the organs are at their minimum volume, the vessels are coiled and stretching just straightens out these coils.

### Vessel radius

Since there is friction between a flowing fluid and the tube in which it is contained, the ratio between the cross-sectional area and the surface area of the tube constitutes a second determinant of resistance. This means that small tubes have higher resistance per unit length than large tubes. Because the critical factor is cross-sectional area rather than radius, resistance changes in proportion to the fourth power of the radius, with the result that only small incremental changes in vessel size confer very large changes in resistance. For example, halving the radius would increase resistance 16-fold.

The fact that resistance is greater in small vessels indicates that absolute resistance must be lower in veins than in arteries, since all segments of veins are around twice the size of the equivalent arterial vessels. The relatively low venous resistance is essential for efficient circulation, since the role of the venous system is simply to drain blood back to the heart as rapidly as possible and is reflected in the fact that the same left cardiac output requires a pressure gradient of around (100–30) or 70 mmHg to deliver it to the capillaries but only (20–0) or 20 mmHg to return it from the capillaries to the heart.

The dependence of resistance on absolute vessel size also indicates that the major component of total peripheral resistance must be localized to the smaller precapillary vessels (the microcirculation) rather than the large distributing arteries. Not only are these microcirculatory vessels smaller in radius but they also branch repeatedly every mm or so. Although total cross-sectional area increases with each branching, total surface area increases even more, so that resistance rises rapidly along quite a short distance.

While most textbooks talk about the arterioles as being the primary site of peripheral resistance, this is an oversimplification. The arterioles are the smallest of the precapillary vessels, with luminal diameters of 200 μm or less, but in fact all the small muscular arteries less than around 1 mm in diameter that give rise to these arterioles also constitute a major source of resistance.

What may appear paradoxical is that the high resistance is restricted to the precapillary vasculature, while systemic capillaries have diameters of around 7 μm and so are rather narrower than even the smallest arteriole, yet impose less resistance to flow. The lower resistance in capillaries than arterioles reflects the fact that several capillaries arise from each arteriole, so that the total capillary cross-sectional area:surface area ratio is very much greater than is associated with any generation of arterioles. In terms of functional efficiency, it is of course essential for local resistance not to limit flow through the capillary bed.

## Blood viscosity

The viscosity of a moving fluid represents the amount of friction between the components of the fluid, in contrast to the friction that occurs by interaction of the fluid with the surrounding tube surface. Any friction will increase the amount of energy that is needed to move a fluid along a tube, so viscosity must constitute a further factor contributing to flow resistance.

Different fluids have very different viscosities – think of water and honey – but all fluids that consist only of molecules in solution have viscosities that remain constant regardless of the velocity of fluid movement. Such solutions are termed Newtonian fluids. By contrast, fluids that contain suspended material (non-Newtonian fluids) have viscosities that vary with flow velocity, being greater at low rates of movement. This property is termed *anomalous viscosity*. Because blood is a suspension of cells in plasma, it behaves in a non-Newtonian fashion and this has several implications.

Figure 5.1 illustrates the processes that underlie anomalous viscosity in the bloodstream. When the blood is flowing relatively fast (A–B), the cellular components travel as a core in the centre of the vessel, surrounded by a cell-free layer of plasma. The cells are oriented so that they travel edge-on, producing minimal friction between the cell layers and between cells and plasma. The viscosity of the blood in this situation is around 50% greater than that of plasma alone. If the flow velocity falls sufficiently then the orientation of the suspension becomes less organized, with some cells starting to rotate and collide with adjacent cells. This process absorbs some of the energy creating the pressure gradient and so viscosity rises (C–D). If flow rate falls even further, the cellular constituents fall out of suspension and form an aggregate

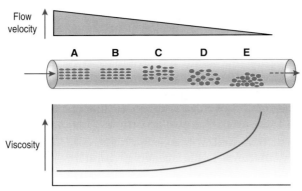

**Figure 5.1** Changes in viscosity and the associated changes in red blood cell behaviour as the velocity of blood flow falls. A & B represent velocities typical of flow in the normal, intact circulation.

on the gravitationally lowest surface of the vessel. Because of the mass of the aggregate, a substantial amount of energy is required to lift the cells back into suspension again, reflected in a very high viscosity (E).

The dependence of blood viscosity on the cellular components has several implications. First, alteration of the haematocrit will change the size of the cell-rich core relative to surrounding plasma. Therefore, increased haematocrit will proportionately elevate viscosity. This can impose a substantial extra cardiac workload particularly during exercise. Thus, 'blood doping' with erythropoietin, although it is likely to improve maximal exercise performance by enhancing oxygen delivery to muscles, also carries a significant risk of damage to the heart. A second consequence of anomalous viscosity is that very low rates of blood flow can result in cells falling out of suspension. If the cell aggregates remain unsuspended for more than a few minutes, they begin to stick together and, in small vessels, may completely obstruct the lumen. This situation is most likely to occur in the postcapillary venules and will be discussed in Chapter 10 in relation to hypotensive states associated with prolonged exercise.

## HANDY HINTS

The width of the cell-free plasma layer is relatively independent of vessel size, because it is dictated by the profiles of the endothelium and the blood cells. By contrast, the number of layers of blood cells that can travel in the cell-rich core must decrease progressively through the microcirculation; in the small arterioles only two or three cells will be able to travel in parallel. With a fall in vessel size, the local blood viscosity must also fall, both because there is reduced friction between the cell core and the surrounding plasma and because there is less friction between adjacent layers of cells. As a result, absolute viscosity in the smallest arterioles may be only about two-thirds that in the aorta.

This has practical implications for measurement of haematocrit during human experiments. Since the usual technique of blood sampling involves finger prick, the origin of the sample is primarily from the superficial microcirculation. It can be predicted that the haematocrit measured in this way is likely to underestimate the true value by at least several per cent and, further, that haematocrit will rise under conditions where the vessels of the finger microcirculation are dilated, such as during heat stress or exercise. Routinely warming the hand in hot water before taking finger prick samples ensures more reproducible and accurate measurements of haematocrit in resting subjects.

Blood flow through systemic capillaries is rather different to that through either precapillary or postcapillary vessels. All these other vessels have diameters greater than that of blood cells, whereas the typical capillary diameter of around 6 μm is marginally less than that of an erythrocytes (8 μm). In consequence, blood cells have to be partially folded in order to pass along the capillary. This process is important in that it ensures the closest contact possible between erythrocyte and endothelial membranes and so minimizes the distance for gas diffusion between blood and tissue. However, in theory it should also produce very high frictional forces between blood cells and the capillary wall, greatly increasing local viscosity and impeding the efficiency of capillary perfusion. To avoid such a disadvantageous situation, the endothelium of capillaries secretes a lubricant mucopolysaccharide that virtually eliminates frictional interaction with the blood cells and results in local viscosity that is almost as low as that of cell-free plasma.

## Poiseuille's law

The equation relating flow, pressure and resistance (see p. 45) can be rewritten by substitution of vessel radius (r) and length (L) and blood viscosity ($V$) for resistance, and adding a factor for numerical accuracy (k), thus:

$$\dot{Q} = k.\Delta P.r^4 / V.L$$

This equation was derived by the scientist Poiseuille and is known as Poiseuille's law. In its full form, with the factor k expressed numerically, it reads:

$$\dot{Q} = 2\Pi.\Delta P.r^4 / 8V.L$$

The practical importance of Poiseuille's law is that it describes the main factors affecting the relationship between flow and pressure. It does not of course take account of homeostatic feedback so does not necessarily predict the end result of manipulating these factors in the whole body. For example, if blood pressure were elevated by a sudden increase in blood volume, there would normally be baroreflex compensation that would lower peripheral resistance and return the pressure to its initial level (see Chapter 7, p. 81). A second difference from the events in the intact circulation is that Poiseuille's law assumes that the vasculature is a system of rigid tubes. As soon as we deal with tubes that might distend in response to internal pressure, then obviously the association between pressure and flow becomes different.

## RESISTANCE TO FLOW OF DISTENSIBLE VESSELS

### Roles of connective tissue and muscle in determining distensibility

In rigid tubes, there is a linear relationship between the pressure gradient and the resulting volume flow, presuming that resistance remains constant (Fig 5.2A). In distensible tubes, by contrast, increased internal pressure will cause some increase in tube volume, so that the rate of volume flow rise with pressure will be lower. In blood vessels, distensibility is conferred by the presence of elastin in the vessel wall, while the presence of collagen confers rigidity (Fig. 5.2B–D). The property of distensibility is usually referred to as *compliance*.

For any given mix of elastin and collagen, absolute vessel compliance depends also on the amount of smooth muscle and whether the muscle cells are relaxed or contracted. Although arterioles have elastin in their walls, they behave as virtually rigid tubes because of the thickness of the muscle layer. The walls of large veins contain large amounts of elastin and relatively small amounts of muscle, so they are normally highly distensible. However, if the muscle contracts fully then this has the effect of stiffening the vein dramatically, so that even high internal pressure does not cause distension.

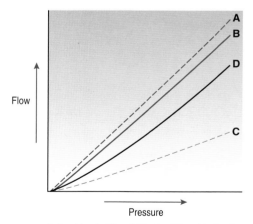

**Figure 5.2** Passive flow–pressure relationships in (A) a rigid tube, (B) an idealized artery in which the wall contains collagen but no elastin, (C) an idealized artery in which the wall contains elastin but no collagen and (D) a typical real artery containing both elastin and collagen.

This transition becomes practically important when one is inserting an intra-venous needle for blood sampling. Unsuccessful insertion frequently causes local muscle spasm in the vein wall, with the result that the vessel shrinks so much that it is impossible to cannulate.

## Measurement of arterial distensibility

The compliance of the arterial system determines the magnitude of arterial pulse pressure, the pulsatility of peripheral blood flow and the velocity of blood flow through the larger arteries. This will in turn affect shear stress on the endothelium and the release of endothelial factors that alter periph-eral resistance (see Chapter 6, p. 64). The arteries become progressively stif-fer with age due to loss of elastin: at any given age higher stiffness is predictive of cardiovascular morbidity, while reduction of blood pressure associated with, for example, chronic exercise programmes is linked to reduced stiffness. Measuring arterial stiffness is, therefore, potentially useful not only for evaluating the basis of circulatory parameters such as blood pressure, but also for assessing cardiovascular health and monitoring the beneficial effects of interventions like exercise.

A number of techniques exist for evaluating arterial stiffness, all of which utilize non-invasive detection of the phasic blood pressure waveform and varying degrees of technology. Conceptually simplest, and the original stan-dard, is measurement of pulse wave velocity by timing arrival of the peak pressure wave at two sites different distances away from the heart, tradition-ally in the carotid and the femoral arteries (Fig. 5.3A). Other methods can utilize pressure waves recorded from one peripheral arterial site (usually

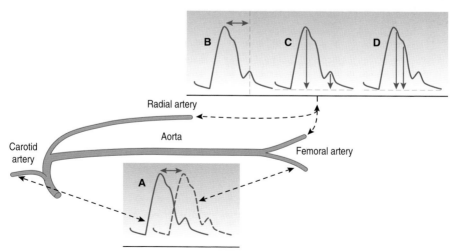

**Figure 5.3** Some of the approaches used for assessment of arterial stiffness from non-invasive analysis of the arterial pulse wave. (A) Pulse wave velocity. (B) Reflection time. (C) Peripheral augmentation index. (D) Central augmentation index.

the femoral or radial) and involve measurement of the time interval between the systolic pressure peak and the reflected wave that follows it (Fig. 5.3B), comparison of the amplitudes of these two events (Fig. 5.3C) or assessment of the shape of the primary systolic pressure waveform (Fig. 5.3D).

All of these methods involve some assumptions about the physics of the circulation and some require significant amounts of computation. For example, the central augmentation index method (Fig. 5.3D) involves a computerized transfer function that estimates the aortic waveform from the shape of a peripheral systolic wave. Comparison of values obtained with a range of methods in healthy subjects and patient groups has indicated that there is relatively poor agreement between different techniques. This is not surprising since some methods use central and some use peripheral arteries: these two types of artery have different wall characteristics and are at very different distances from reflection sites in the peripheral microcirculation. Optimal assessment of arterial wall behaviour should, therefore, employ more than one technique, so as to involve both vessel types. However, it remains to be determined which combination of methods is most useful. For the present, the choice is based primarily on what facilities are available in particular laboratories.

## EFFECT OF INTRAVASCULAR PRESSURE ON WALL TENSION

In the intact circulation, blood vessels are always subject to outwardly exerted pressure. This imposes tension on the structural elements of the vessel wall that have the potential to cause vessel rupture. The amount of tension generated by a particular transmural pressure ($\Delta P$) depends both on the luminal radius (r) and on the thickness of the vessel wall (w) and the relationship between these factors is expressed in Laplace's law:

$$\text{Tension} = \Delta P.r/w$$

## Laplace's law and large vessel function

In rigid tubes, it is clear that wall tension is independent of intravascular pressure. If the tube is distensible, by contrast, increased intravascular pressure will not only increase r, but also reduce w, so that wall tension rises rapidly. With the magnitudes of pressure and vessel size characteristic of the aorta during systolic ejection, increases in vessel radius by around 50% would be likely to cause wall rupture. The protection against this is the presence of a non-distensible layer of collagen fibres around the aorta. These are arranged so that they allow aortic radius to increase by about 20% during systolic ejection, consistent with its function in facilitating diastolic flow (see Chapter 4, p. 31), but form a rigid outer sleeve to the vessel that prevents further increases in radius (Fig 5.4). Although this protective mechanism is highly

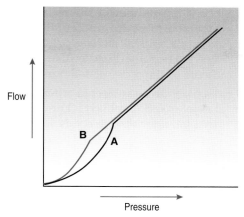

**Figure 5.4** Pressure–flow relationship in the aorta. (A) The collagen elements of the wall are arranged so as to allow some distension but when this reaches its limits the collagen behaves like a rigid sheath. (B) When the aortic smooth muscle is contracted, this tightens the collagen matrix and reduces distensibility. Note that under these conditions a given value of flow is achieved at a lower pressure.

effective, it can be disrupted in people with pathologies that cause selective loss of collagen from the body. If these individuals are subject to sudden rises in blood pressure, they may, therefore, experience uncontrolled aortic distension leading to wall rupture (a *dissecting aneurysm*) and potentially fatal haemorrhage.

Laplace's law is not important for venous integrity, because the relatively low intravascular pressures do not produce significant wall tension. The large veins, therefore, do not require restrictive collagen layers in their walls and are able to distend to several times their resting diameters in their role as blood storage reservoirs.

## Laplace's law and small vessel function

In the precapillary microcirculation, although intravascular pressure is of the same order of magnitude as in the aorta, the luminal size is too small for absolute wall tension to ever reach values that might cause wall damage. In these small arterial vessels, Laplace's law has functional significance of another sort. The walls of small arteries and arterioles contain little connective tissue and consist primarily of smooth muscle that usually has some degree of active tone – that is, is in a state of partial contraction – due to sympathetic vasoconstrictor nerve activity and circulating vasoconstrictor hormones. Under these circumstances, the vessel luminal size must reflect a balance between the outwardly directed pressure of the blood and the inwardly directed pressure exerted by the muscle. If intravascular pressure falls suddenly, then the vessel will constrict without opposition down to a minimal luminal diameter. The absolute pressure necessary to balance muscle tone is termed the *critical closing pressure*, and imposes a further modification on the relationship between pressure and flow, since it means that in the microcirculation flow ceases while there is still a measurable pressure gradient (Fig. 5.5). In arterioles with high vasoconstrictor tone, the critical closing pressure may be as great as 60–70 mmHg. If the vessels are fully dilated, then flow would persist with very low pressure gradients of the order of 4–5 mmHg.

The vessel segment most likely to be subject to critical closure is the region of transition between arteriole and capillary, known as the metarteriole, because within the muscular arteriolar tree this last region is the smallest in diameter and has least supporting tissue. The relationship between contractile state and metarteriolar closure is an important determinant of blood flow distribution in tissues, such as skeletal muscle, and will be discussed further in the next chapter (pp. 69–73).

## MEASUREMENT OF PERIPHERAL BLOOD FLOW

In animal studies, a range of methodologies is available for accurate measurement of regional blood flows and vascular properties, and a large proportion of the information that we have on control of peripheral blood flow comes from these data. However, the techniques used in animal experiments are in general more invasive than is practicable for human studies. This next section will survey the techniques that are used routinely in human experiments, focusing on measurement of parameters that are important in studies of exercise, and summarize their relative advantages and limitations.

### Temperature

Skin temperature reflects a balance between the rate at which heat arrives from the body core in the cutaneous blood supply and the rate at which this

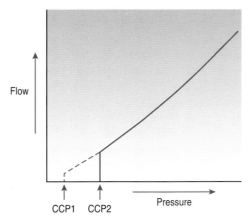

**Figure 5.5** Flow–pressure relationship in an arteriole. The arteriolar wall behaves almost like a rigid tube because of its thick smooth muscle coat, but flow ceases due to vessel closure when perfusion pressure falls below a critical pressure (critical closing pressure, CCP).

heat is lost into the environment. Provided that the local environmental conditions can be controlled, therefore, skin temperature is often used as a semi-quantitative index of skin blood flow. The main advantage of this technique is that it can provide moment-to-moment indicators of skin perfusion over a wide area of the body surface, making it useful, for example, for evaluating cutaneous vasomotor responses to thermoregulatory stimuli. Aside from the obvious fact that no calibration of flow is possible, other limitations of this technique include the need to prevent interference from sweat-induced evaporative heat loss and the fact that high metabolic rates of underlying tissues, such as muscle, may distort the temperature recorded at the skin surface.

## Pulse transduction

The haemoglobin content of red blood cells means that they differentially reflect electromagnetic radiation frequencies that pass through the other tissue constituents. Since the absolute volume of red blood cells within a tissue varies proportionately with blood flow, this provides a method by which pulsatile blood flow can be visualized and, to some extent, the level of flow assessed. In human experimentation, the application of these pulse transduction techniques is for monitoring of skin blood flow. In relatively thin tissues, such as fingers and ear lobe, red light can be shone through the tissue and detected using a photoelectric cell on the opposite side. Measurement of superficial blood flow in other areas can be achieved by detection of reflected light with photoelectric elements adjacent to the light emitter or by measuring the Doppler shift in frequency of the reflected beam.

With all these devices, pulsatile signal amplitude rises with cutaneous arteriolar dilation and so is roughly proportional to blood flow. The devices that rely on photoelectric detection, however, have the limitation that no calibration of flow is possible. By contrast, the more sophisticated devices that utilize Doppler shift detection and which involve laser light sources, have inbuilt algorithms that allow estimation of zero flow and so can be calibrated. Pulse transduction cannot be used for measurement of muscle blood flow because the path length of the practicable light sources is insufficient to penetrate that far below the skin.

## Venous occlusion plethysmography

If venous outflow from a tissue is obstructed, the continued arterial inflow will initially produce an equivalent increase in tissue volume. At the same time, intravascular pressure in the tissue capillaries and veins rises progressively towards arterial pressure. When venous pressure reaches the occluding pressure then venous outflow is re-established and no further increase in tissue volume occurs. Provided that the tissue involved is able to swell in response to arterial inflow for at least a few heart beats, which is the case for most tissues, then the volume change gives an accurate measurement of regional blood flow.

In practice, this technique of measuring volume change (*plethysmography*) in response to venous occlusion is usually applied to measurement of limb blood flow, and then most commonly to that in forearm. The subject is seated with the forearm in a horizontal position and at or slightly above the level of the heart. An occlusive cuff is applied to the upper arm and inflated repetitively for periods of several seconds to a pressure above that in the arm veins but below diastolic arterial pressure – this pressure is typically set at 40 mmHg and the inflation–deflation cycle is typically of the order of 4 s–6 s. Tissue volume is quantified from arm circumference, measured by a stretchable strain gauge wrapped around the midpoint of the forearm. Without cuff inflation, it is usually possible to observe small pulsatile changes in arm circumference with every pulse wave (Fig. 5.6). Cuff inflation causes a progressive rise in circumference that becomes less pronounced after the first few heart beats as venous pressure rises and will plateau after some seconds when venous pressure exceeds the cuff pressure. Flow is calculated by measuring the gradient of the early, steepest part of the curve and converting this to the rate of volume change of the tissue slice beneath the strain gauge (Fig. 5.6).

Because the distensible tissues of the forearm consist of both muscle and skin, venous occlusion plethysmography measures blood flow through both and interpretation of the vascular bed responsible for experimentally induced flow changes is based largely on the situation. For example, skin perfusion can be held at a low and stable level by maintaining a cool environment and hyperaemia following brief isometric forearm exercise must by definition be primarily localized to muscle. By contrast, increases in flow

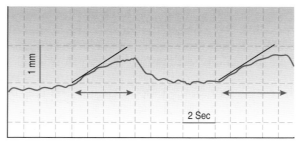

1 mm

2 Sec

**Figure 5.6** Venous occlusion plethysmography of the forearm. Periods of cuff inflation are denoted by the horizontal arrows. During the periods between inflation, pulsatile changes in arm circumference are associated with each cardiac cycle. Note that during inflation the first few cardiac cycles are associated with a rapid rise in circumference but that this plateaus as venous pressure in the arm rises. Blood flow is measured from the rate of rise in circumference during the first two cardiac cycles of the inflation period, as indicated by the red lines. Initial forearm circumference was 200 mm, so its radius was 32 mm, and the strain gauge covered a 1 mm length of arm. The initial tissue volume at the measurement site was therefore $\Pi$. $32^2$ or 3215 mm$^3$, approximating to 3.2 g tissue. Venous occlusion caused swelling by 1 mm circumference (0.16 mm radius)/4 s, equating to a volume change of 33 mm$^3$/4 s or 495 mm$^3$/min per 3.3 g tissue, which corresponds to 0.495 mL/min/3.3 or 15 mL/min/100 g.

associated specifically with body warming can be assumed to occur primarily in skin. For accurate assessment of skin blood-flow responses to thermal stimuli it is preferable to measure not only forearm, but also finger blood flow, because the fingers are devoid of muscle. As well, since the finger circulation contains arteriovenous shunts (see Chapter 5, p. 60), simultaneous monitoring of arm and finger flows sometimes provides differential information on the responses of shunt and arteriolar vessels to thermal stimuli.

Finger volume is measured in an identical way to that used for forearm. Some investigators favour placement of the occlusive cuff at the wrist on the basis that leaving the whole forearm venous supply intact damps the rate of finger swelling: on the other hand, the initial inflation artefact is much larger when using a wrist cuff and this can lead to inaccuracy of flow measurement. On balance, this author recommends retaining the cuff on the upper arm.

Similar principles are used for measurement of leg blood flow, but in a standing posture the gravitational forces result in venous distension and high intra-tissue pressure that may interfere with volume changes during venous occlusion. Greater accuracy is, therefore, assured if the subject is sitting or lying.

## Doppler imaging

Positioning a pulsed Doppler transducer over a relatively superficial artery allows the velocity of blood flow at that site to be quantified. An adjacent Doppler head can provide an image of the arterial diameter, so together these pieces of information can be transcribed into absolute volume flow. This technique can be used on the brachial artery to measure blood flow to the forearm or on the femoral artery to measure blood flow to the leg. However, the need to have extremely accurate placement of the Doppler heads makes it possible to measure flow during exercise only if the limb segment involved is immobilized. Thus, for leg exercise, only movements of the lower leg are possible.

## Thermal dilution

If a known amount of an indicator (in this case, cold) is introduced into the arterial blood supply, then it will appear at a more distal part of the vascular bed at a rate that reflects the volume flow. This technique is used routinely in some exercise laboratories that are skilled in invasive procedures, for measurement of leg blood flow. The radial artery is cannulated in the groin and a bolus of cold saline is injected. The rate at which this cold fluid travels through the leg circulation is determined by a thermistor placed in the femoral vein and an algorithm allows calculation of volume flow. Since no movement artefacts occur, this technique is compatible with even high intensity whole-body exercise and the accuracy is high. However, the invasive nature of the procedure obviously restricts its application.

## STRUCTURAL SPECIALIZATION OF BLOOD VESSELS

Two situations exist in which structural specialization of blood vessels provides unique functional properties that are not found in most vascular beds. One of these is the parallel arrangement of arterial and venous vessels that provides an opportunity for recycling of material between arterial and venous blood. The other is a system of wide, low-resistance vessels that allow blood to be shunted from arterial to venous circulations without transiting the capillaries.

## Countercurrent exchangers

When the arterial and venous limbs of a circulatory bed are closely apposed to each other, two streams of blood travel parallel to each other but in opposite directions. Under these circumstances, any substance that is in a higher concentration in one limb tends to diffuse down its concentration gradient into the other limb. If the higher concentration is in the arterial blood then some substance is returned into the venous bloodstream rather than reaching the capillaries: if the higher concentration is in the venous blood then some will be recycled into the arterial stream rather than travelling on into the central veins.

Different types of substance can be exchanged in these counter-current loops dependent on whether the loop involves large or microcirculatory vessels. Thermal energy diffuses rapidly over quite long distances through body tissues, so heat can easily be transferred between large arteries and veins. By contrast, solute exchange can occur only in the microcirculation because molecular diffusion is efficient only over distances of a few microns.

### *Countercurrent heat exchange*

Countercurrent exchange of heat in large vessels is an essential part of thermoregulation since it is used to vary the amount of core body heat that is lost into the environment. A large fraction of total heat exchange takes place in the hands and feet and especially in the digits. These are sites of very large surface area:volume ratio and afford a large area for exchange and a relatively efficient pathway for diffusion of heat from bloodstream to skin surface. This can be used to optimize heat loss under conditions of heat stress or exercise by removal of sympathetic vasoconstrictor tone to the limb vessels, which both increases extremity blood flow and ensures that the venous drainage from these areas travels in veins close to the skin surface.

When the body is exposed to a cold environment, by contrast, then even the relatively small volume of blood reaching the extremities under vasoconstricted conditions loses a lot of its internal heat and places an additional metabolic load on the body if core body temperature is to remain stable. For metabolic economy it is, therefore, sensible to minimize heat loss in the extremities. This is achieved by sympathetic changes in venous tone that divert drainage in the limbs to deep veins lying adjacent to the main arteries. In this situation, heat is transferred from arterial to venous blood as it travels down the limbs, and recycled back into the central circulation (Fig. 5.7A).

## Countercurrent solute exchange

Microcirculatory countercurrent exchange of solutes is functionally important in two regions – the epithelium of the small intestine and the vasa recta of the renal medulla. In each of these situations, the actual vascular organization consists of a quite complex network of vessels but can be envisaged, in simplified form, as a hairpin loop consisting of an arteriole leading to a capillary loop and then a venule that runs parallel and close to the arteriole. By definition, the concentration of oxygen is higher in arterial than in venous plasma, so some incoming arterial oxygen always diffuses across into the parallel stream of venous blood along the length of the loop. Thus, the tissue cells near the loop end are always living in a relatively hypoxic environment even at high total rates of organ blood flow (Fig. 5.7A). These cells are, therefore, unusually susceptible to damage if local blood flow falls. Exchange in the opposite direction will occur with any solutes that are taken up into the capillary loop from the interstitium and so are in higher concentration in the venous than the arterial plasma (Fig. 5.7B). This applies in the intestine to any absorbed nutrients and in the renal medulla to the urea and sodium that have been concentrated by selective movement out of the distal nephron. The result of this countercurrent exchange is to recycle solute from the venous into the arterial plasma and so limit the amount of solute entering the venous return. In the intestine, this ensures that absorbed nutrients do not reach the liver faster than they can be processed and stored. In the kidney, it provides a mechanism for retention of the medullary interstitial hyperosmolarity that is essential for regulation of urinary water loss.

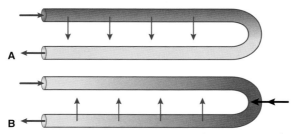

**Figure 5.7** Countercurrent exchange between an arterial and a venous vessel in parallel. In (A), material entering in the arterial bloodstream (dark shading) is partially lost into the venous return before it reaches the most distal portion of the vascular bed. In (B), material diffusing into the capillaries forming the end of the loop (dark shading) is partially recycled through the loop, slowing the rate of venous clearance.

## Arteriovenous shunts

In the previous section we saw that the digits are a major site of heat loss from the body because of their large surface area:volume ratios. A similar thermo-regulatory function is served by other small superficial tissues with large sur-face areas, the ears and the nose. In all these tissues, heat exchange is optimized further by the presence of short, large diameter vessels that connect large arterioles directly to large venules, bypassing the resistance of the smal-ler arterioles. These so-called *arteriovenous anastomoses* or *shunts* have thick walls containing circular bands of smooth muscle, which can shut off the lumen of the vessel entirely when contracted. Under those conditions, all flow takes place through capillaries. If the shunt muscle is relaxed, the low resis-tance of the shunt vessels means that total blood flow to these areas of the skin rises dramatically. Like other vascular smooth muscles, the shunt muscle receives a sympathetic innervation and, therefore, the withdrawal of sympa-thetic tone to the skin circulation that occurs during during body heating not only increases skin blood flow generally but in addition opens up the shunts.

The shunt vessels subserve a second thermoregulatory function in that they open not only during heat stress but also when local skin temperature reaches a value just above freezing point. At these local temperatures, therefore, blood flow through the fingers, toes, ears and nose suddenly rises dramati-cally from the low values that are characteristic of skin perfusion during sym-pathetic vasoconstriction (Fig. 5.8). This response, termed *cold vasodilatation*, is potentially important for preventing freezing of peripheral tissues that cool down particularly rapidly. While this role imposes a significant extra thermal load on the body because it involves loss of additional body heat into the

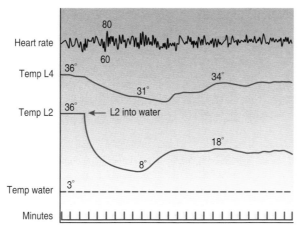

**Figure 5.8** Skin temperatures recorded from the plantar surfaces of second and fourth fingers of the left hand (L2, L4) during immersion of L2 in water at 3°C for 20 min. Note that the immersed finger begins to rewarm once skin temperature falls below 8°C and that the temperature is subsequently maintained at 16–18°C. Note also that the temperature oscillation is not restricted to the immersed finger. From Bell & Robbins (1997), reproduced with permission of the publishers.

environment, this is minimized for the limbs, where total flow and, therefore, potential heat loss is highest, by the countercurrent recycling of arterial heat into the deep veins (see Countercurrent heat exchange, above).

The mechanism of cold vasodilatation is not well understood. Smooth muscle cells lose their contractile ability when they are cooled below about 10°C, so shunt opening could be due to this cold-induced paralysis overriding the constrictor effect of sympathetic nerve activity. Some data, however, suggest that this is too simplistic an explanation. For one thing, the increased local blood flow that accompanies shunt opening can rewarm the skin to values considerably above those that cause muscle paralysis, but this is not always followed by another bout of shunt closure and recooling. As well, when cooling is restricted to one digit, less exaggerated increases in blood flow occur synchronously in adjacent fingers (Fig. 5.8). Finally, some studies have reported deficits in cold vasodilatation in limbs with damaged innervation and noted that the response normalized as nerve regeneration took place. Together, these findings suggest that the cold vasodilator response may involve activation of dilator nerves rather than being a purely local phenomenon.

## Key points

For a given perfusion pressure gradient, blood flow is affected by blood viscosity and by the behaviour of the vessel walls.

In large arterial vessels, the connective tissue components of the wall make resistance less than that of a rigid tube, while in the microcirculation the smooth muscle coat makes the vessels virtually non-distensible.

Several indices of arterial stiffness are available, but it is likely that these provide information on the behaviour of different segments of the arterial tree.

The choice between available techniques for measurement of limb muscle and skin blood depends primarily on the temporal and quantitative accuracy needed. With most, movement artefacts restrict measurement during exercise.

Countercurrent exchange between large arteries and veins of the limbs provides an essential way of reducing body heat loss in cold environments. Countercurrent exchange in microcirculatory beds provides a mechanism for regulating solute movement between bloodstream and interstitium.

Arteriovenous shunts are an important site of body heat transfer between bloodstream and skin, and provide a valuable mechanism for preventing cold damage to the extremities.

## Reference

Bell C, Robbins S 1997 Autonomic vasodilatation in the skin. In: Morris JH, Gibbins IL (eds) Autonomic Innervation of the Skin. Harwood, Amsterdam, pp. 87–110.

## Further reading

Berne RM, Levy MN 2001 Hemodynamics. In: Cardiovascular Physiology, 8th edn. Mosby, St Louis.
Panerai RB 2003 The critical closing pressure of the cerebral circulation. Medical Engineering and Physics 25: 621–632.
Woodman RJ, Kingwell BA, Beilin LJ, Hamilton SE, Dart AM, Watts G 2005 Assessment of central and peripheral arterial stiffness: studies indicating the need to use a combination of techniques. American Journal of Hypertension 18: 249–260.

### Questions for revision

- Why does the viscosity of blood vary with flow velocity?
- Why does the haematocrit of blood sampled from a finger-tip vary depending on whether the finger is warm or cold?
- What is the significance of Laplace's law for the function of (a) large arteries and (b) arterioles?
- What is the equation that describes Poiseuille's law?
- What applications are made of the Doppler shift in measurement of peripheral arterial function?
- Discuss the advantages and limitations of different techniques for quantifying limb blood flow.
- Discuss the functional importance of countercurrent exchange in blood vessels.

Chapter **6**

# Local regulation of vascular function

## CHAPTER CONTENTS

### After reading this chapter, you should be able to:

- identify the endothelial factors that contribute to regulation of regional blood flows and the techniques available for assessing endothelial function

- understand how local metabolites contribute to regulation of regional blood flows

- know the basis of local myogenic regulation of vascular resistance

- describe the roles of these various local influences in autoregulation, vasomotion and functional hyperaemia of exercise

Even in the absence of unusual structural design features like those discussed at the end of the last chapter, there is not always a straightforward relationship between regional microcirculatory blood flow and the applied pressure gradient. In many tissues, changes in perfusion pressure do not cause corresponding changes in flow because local adjustments of microcirculatory resistance tend to maintain blood flow constant (*autoregulation*). In addition, in some tissues with relatively low metabolic rates the blood flow is distributed unevenly across the capillary bed, with intermittent perfusion of capillaries in different areas (*vasomotion*). Finally, local vascular conductance is proportional to local tissue metabolism, with increased metabolic rate causing vasodilation and increased blood flow (*functional hyperaemia*). These three phenomena are due to a mixture of factors, the most universally important of which are the local vasodilator actions of chemicals released from the endothelium, local metabolites and the response of vascular smooth muscle cells to altered transmural pressure.

We will first examine the mechanisms involved in each of these three categories of local control.

## ENDOTHELIAL CONTROL OF LOCAL CONDUCTANCE

### Identity of endothelium-derived vasoactive factors

Endothelial cells release several factors that affect vascular smooth muscle cell activity. The most studied of these is the vasodilator nitric oxide (NO), endothelial synthesis of which is dependent on free intracellular $Ca^{2+}$. NO acts by diffusing into the muscle cells and activating guanylate cyclase. There is good evidence that continual release of NO from the endothelium leads to a tonic dilator effect on the vascular smooth muscle, the magnitude of which depends on the balance between rate of release and rate of dispersal into the bloodstream. In addition, increased shear stress on the endothelium increases NO release. This probably constitutes an important factor in regulation of vessel calibre in large conduit arteries (see Chapter 7, p. 81) but, because of the large total cross-sectional area and concomitant low flow velocity in microvascular beds, the effect of shear stress on release of endothelial mediators in arterioles is likely to be much less substantial.

A second group of endothelium-derived dilator (or relaxing) factors (EDRFs) is the prostaglandins (PGs). Endothelial PG synthesis is regulated by the availability of the precursor arachidonic acid, the intracellular level of which is elevated by increased free intracellular $Ca^{2+}$ and by shear stress. Thus, the factors that affect endothelial PG release are similar to those affecting NO release. Although the available evidence suggests that PGs serve a less important role than does NO in tonic modulation of vascular resistance, prostacyclin ($PGI_2$) in particular has been implicated in some dilator processes (see Functional hyperaemia during exercise, below).

A number of additional biologically active factors of endothelial origin also exist, including EDRFs, that causes muscle cell hyperpolarization (endothelium-derived hyperpolarizing factor, EDHF) and for which there are several candidate molecules, together with the endothelins that cause vasoconstriction. None of these factors have been studied to the same extent as NO and their physiological significance is not yet clear, but it seems probable that at least collectively they may play a significant role in regulation of peripheral resistance (Quyyumi & Ozkor 2006).

# Assessment of endothelial control of local conductance

## *Reactive hyperaemia*

If the arterial inflow to a tissue is occluded for more than a few seconds, the conduit and microcirculatory arterial vessels dilate downstream of the occlusion. As a result, release of the occlusion is accompanied by a temporary elevation of local blood flow above the pre-occlusion level, termed *reactive hyperaemia*. The reactive hyperaemic responses of both conduit and microcirculatory vessels are attenuated after administration of substances that prevent NO production, suggesting that both involve EDRFs and might, therefore, be utilized as indices of endothelial dilator function. It is uncertain whether EDRFs other than NO are implicated.

Reactive hyperaemia is usually elicited in the forearm with occlusion of the brachial artery above the elbow for a period of between 2 and 3 min. In these circumstances, the peak flow immediately after release of occlusion is typically two to four times the pre-occlusion value and returns to this resting level over 30–50 s. Conduit vessel dilation is assessed using ultrasound imaging of brachial artery diameter, and the reactive hyperaemic response is referred to as *flow-mediated dilation*. Microcirculatory dilation is usually assessed either by measurement of blood flow through forearm or finger using venous occlusion plethysmography (Fig. 6.1) or by laser-Doppler measurement of forearm skin flow.

Comparative studies show poor correlation between the magnitudes of large and small vessel responses in different subject populations (Hansell et al 2004), which is perhaps not surprising if we consider the mechanisms likely to underlie dilation in the two vessel types. Assuming that all endothelial cells release EDRFs continuously, local accumulation of these factors during the period of arterial occlusion should have similar dilator consequences in large and small vessels once the normal pressure gradient is re-established. In conduit vessels, however, the increased volume flow will be accompanied

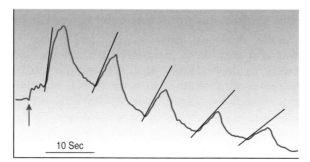

**Figure 6.1** Venous occlusion plethysmographic record of forearm blood flow immediately following cessation (at red arrow) of 3 min brachial arterial occlusion. The red lines indicate rates of rise of tissue circumference during each period of venous occlusion. Note the high initial reactive hyperaemia and the subsequent decline in blood flow over the succeeding minute. From Barry (2003) with permission of the author.

by a high rate of shear stress on the endothelium that will increase local EDRF release further. As flow velocity is much lower in the microcirculation, shear stress is not likely to generate factor release at that site. A second complicating factor arises from the fact that cessation of blood flow through a tissue results in local accumulation of dilator metabolites (see Chapter 6, p. 67). Depending on the metabolic rate of the tissue and the duration of arterial occlusion, metabolic dilation in the microcirculation may, therefore, act additively with EDRFs.

It is not certain at present whether reactive hyperaemia in large or in small arteries provides the better index of physiological endothelial behaviour. Purely from the point of view that the microcirculation contributes to peripheral resistance most, it seems logical that this site should be used if the investigators' concern is the implications of endothelial function for blood pressure control. If one adopts this position, then it is clearly essential to avoid interference by endothelium-independent metabolic dilation. Given the fact that skin metabolism is negligible unless there is active sweating, using skin rather than whole forearm blood flow may provide more accurate data.

## Endothelial turnover

The endothelium is turning over continually, with dying cells being shed into the circulation and being replaced by new cells that originate from circulating bone marrow-derived progenitors. These processes may provide additional indices by which the functional status of the endothelium can be assessed at a whole-body level. On the one hand, large numbers of dislodged endothelial cells in the blood stream could indicate reduced viability, consistent with reduced EDRF function. A number of studies have reported elevated numbers of circulating endothelial cells (CECs) in various disease states associated with other evidence of reduced endothelial dilator capacity, including hypertension and diabetes. Conversely, it could be argued that rapid cell turnover would lower the average age of the endothelial population and so reduce the proportion of old, metabolically sub-optimal cells. This possibility is consistent with observations that CECs rise in parallel with endothelial dilator capacity in healthy subjects during aerobic training (see Chapter 11, p. 134).

CEC numbers alone, therefore, provide only ambiguous information on endothelial status and additional markers of endothelial viability must be used concomitantly in order to decide whether high CEC values denote healthy or unhealthy endothelium. One marker that may be useful is Von Willebrand factor, which is released from endothelial cells in response to inflammatory stimuli. Von Willebrand factor levels appear to be elevated in at least most pathological situations where CEC numbers are increased. By contrast, the one study that has compared these parameters with fitness levels in healthy subjects (O'Sullivan 2003) found that the rise in CECs associated with training was not linked to any change in plasma Von Willebrand levels.

## Assessment of nitric-oxide involvement in endothelial control of local conductance

### Release of nitric oxide

It can be anticipated that NO released from endothelium will diffuse into the bloodstream as well as into the vascular wall, so that plasma levels of NO could provide an index of endothelial dilator function. Detection of NO itself is not practicable, since the NO molecule is metabolized too rapidly to allow blood sampling and assay. However, the main breakdown product of NO, nitrite ion, is stable and recent studies have demonstrated good correlation between serum nitrite levels and other markers of NO-dependent dilation (Rassaf et al 2006).

### Responses to dilator agonists

The most specific technique for quantifying the ability of endothelial cells to release NO involves comparison of vascular responses to a dilator agonist that acts by releasing endothelial NO (typically acetylcholine) with responses to a NO donor that acts directly on the smooth muscle (typically sodium nitroprusside). However, in order to avoid reflex changes in sympathetic vascular tone complicating the results, it is necessary to be able to administer the dilator agonists in low concentration, directly into a regional arterial bed. Thus, invasive arterial cannulation is required, making the technique unsuitable for many research applications.

## METABOLIC CONTROL OF LOCAL CONDUCTANCE

All known cellular metabolites, including adenosine nucleotide degradation products, $CO_2$, phosphates, lactate and protons, have dilator actions on vascular smooth muscle. This provides a mechanism by which local vascular conductance can, in theory, be matched automatically to tissue metabolic demands. At least some of the activity of certain metabolites (for example adenine molecules) is produced via their stimulating release of NO and other endothelial dilator factors; other metabolites, such as protons, appear to act directly on the vascular smooth muscle. Since the balance between different factors depends on the precise metabolic pathways utilized in a tissue, the dilator contributions of each metabolite vary between different organ systems. Identifying the relative importance of different factors in particular situations may be important since variations in those factors that are most potent, or in highest concentration, may be the most reliable index of hyperaemia. Because of this, much debate has taken place in the research literature as regards the roles of specific factors in, for example skeletal muscle (Clifford & Hellsten 2004).

In terms of functional significance, on the other hand, the evidence to date suggests that no single identified factor is overwhelmingly important in any tissue (see Functional hyperaemia during exercise, p. 72, for further discussion). This does not necessarily imply that another unknown factor is the main contributor. The non-specificity of functional dilatation can be ascribed partly to the additive dilator effects of all metabolites present. It also reflects the fact that absolute interstitial osmolality is a powerful vaso-dilator influence regardless of the identity of the osmotically active particles. In addition, it is possible that certain metabolites may have far greater biological efficacy when present at the outer surface of the vascular media than when presented in the bloodstream as is common in experimental studies.

The effect of metabolites is amplified in some tissues by several other vasodi-lator influences that are proportional in intensity to tissue activity. The most widespread of these is mediated by a population of ion channels on vascular smooth muscle cells that open in response to locally reduced dissolved oxygen tension; that is, that function as hypoxia receptors (Quayle et al 2006). Opening of these channels results in cell hyperpolarization and relaxa-tion, so falls in interstitial oxygenation following increased tissue oxygen consumption have a similar effect to that of increased metabolite accumula-tion. Interestingly, the hypoxia receptors in pulmonary arterioles produce local vasoconstriction rather than dilatation, a feature that is very important in regulation of gas exchange in the lung (see Chapter 8, p. 96).

Additional dilator factors are liberated during metabolic activity from par-ticular tissue cell types. These include potassium ions, NO and PGs in the case of striated muscle, short-chain peptides termed kinins in the case of exocrine glands and secretomotor peptide hormones in the case of the gas-trointestinal tract. Further information on these factors and how they may interact during the circulatory adjustments to exercise will be found in the section Functional hyperaemia during exercise, p. 72.

## MYOGENIC CONTROL OF LOCAL CONDUCTANCE

Stretching a vascular smooth muscle cell causes graded depolarization of the cell membrane and this opens voltage-dependent calcium channels. As a result, the level of free intracellular $Ca^{2+}$ rises and the cell contracts; a phe-nomenon known as the *myogenic response*. Experimental studies using isolated arterial segments suggest that the amount of membrane stretch in arterioles due to normal levels of intravascular pressure depolarizes the cells by 20–30 mV, which is sufficient to cause 40–50% constriction relative to their passive diameter (Dora 2005). Thus, a substantial proportion of ongoing total periph-eral resistance related to blood pressure maintenance is due to the myogenic response, independent of vasoconstrictor influences by sympathetic nerves or circulating hormones.

As well as contributing to resting peripheral resistance, the myogenic response is elicited whenever intravascular pressure changes. An increase in arterial perfusion pressure will result in depolarization and arteriolar constriction and, conversely, decreased perfusion pressure will cause hyperpolarization and dilation. The molecular details of the process that monitors membrane distortion are still unclear. The end-result, however, is that the contractile state of the cell does not alter to maintain a stable vessel diameter in the face of altered perfusion pressure. Rather, increased pressure results in a net decrease in diameter and decreased pressure in a net increase. This implies that what is being monitored is not membrane distortion itself, but wall stress.

## AUTOREGULATION

From the pressure/flow relationships discussed in Chapter 5, you would expect changes in perfusion pressure gradient through a regional vascular bed to produce approximately proportionate changes in blood flow. In skeletal and cardiac muscles, brain, gastrointestinal tract and kidney, however, this occurs only with extremely low or high pressures. Over the range typical of most normal circumstances (from somewhere around 60–70 mmHg up to around 150 mmHg) flow changes transiently when pressure is altered but returns over 20–60 s to its previous value, so that flow is effectively independent of pressure over this so-called *autoregulatory* pressure range (Fig. 6.2).

Clearly, maintenance of flow in the face of altered pressure requires adjustment of vascular resistance. The relationships between perfusion pressure and release of endothelial dilator factors, tissue metabolite production and myogenic responses, as discussed above, suggest that any or all of these processes could provide the basis for the autoregulatory response.

In cardiac and skeletal muscles, brain and gastrointestinal tract, changes in local metabolite concentration appear to be the dominant mechanism. At any

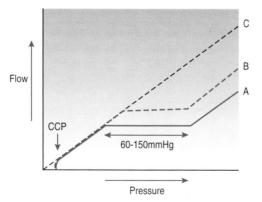

**Figure 6.2** In a microcirculatory vascular bed that exhibits autoregulation, flow remains constant over a range of perfusion pressures that is typically around 60–150 mmHg (A). The absolute value at which flow is regulated is dependent on tissue metabolic rate, with moderately increased metabolism causing increased flow without altering the autoregulatory range (B). At pressures outside the autoregulatory range, the pressure–flow relationship approaches that in rigid tubes (C), unless pressure falls below the critical closing pressure (CCP).

time, absolute microvascular resistance reflects the ambient metabolite concentration. This is a balance between metabolite production and the rate at which these molecules are being washed out of the tissue by the blood flow. If perfusion pressure is altered, the rate of washout will change, resulting in accumulation of metabolites and reduced vascular resistance if perfusion pressure falls or depletion of metabolites and vasoconstriction if pressure rises.

It is uncertain to what extent endothelial and myogenic processes participate in the autoregulatory response in muscle, brain and digestive tract in vivo. Both are well suited to the task: the myogenic response involves identical effects of perfusion pressure on vascular resistance, as does autoregulation, and the scenario outlined above for the effects of altered blood flow on metabolite washout could be postulated to apply equally to washout of endothelium-derived dilator factors, such as NO. These processes may contribute to the rapidity of autoregulatory adjustments, but are unlikely to be essential to autoregulatory responses in the tissues listed above, since these all have relatively high metabolic rates and, therefore, the interstitial levels of metabolites are subject to rapid change in the face of altered perfusion.

The renal circulation also exhibits powerful autoregulation. Here, however, autoregulation is needed not to maintain metabolism, but because a high blood flow is needed for continual removal of waste products from the bloodstream. Since this rate of blood flow is far in excess of the metabolic needs of the renal tissue, metabolites could not transduce the autoregulatory signal. It is thought that renal autoregulation relies primarily on the myogenic response and, consistent with this, the latency of renal resistance responses to altered perfusion pressure is considerably faster (less than 20 s) than is seen typically in other autoregulating vascular beds.

## VASOMOTION

Although autoregulation can maintain stable total organ blood flow despite altered perfusion pressure, provided that metabolic rate remains constant, this does not necessarily mean that the organ is perfused evenly. When the tissue cells are inactive, as in resting skeletal muscles, blood flow may be so low that intravascular pressure within the microcirculation is not sufficient to prevent some arteriolar vessels collapsing under the constraints of Laplace's law (see Chapter 5, p. 52). Under these circumstances there is intermittent perfusion of neighbouring portions of the capillary bed, a process known as *vasomotion*.

The phenomenon of vasomotion relies on the fact that absolute critical closing pressure (CCP) is inversely related to the local concentration of interstitial metabolites. The sequence of events involved is most easily visualized by simplifying the vasculature to one arteriole giving rise to two sequential metarterioles and capillaries (Fig. 6.3) (in real life, three or more sequential metarterioles would be present). Imagine that, initially, the interstitial metabolite concentration is homogenous so that both metarterioles have similar CCPs. That which is more distally located along the parent arteriole will be most likely to close, since perfusion pressure must be lower in that region. A situation will, therefore, be created where the

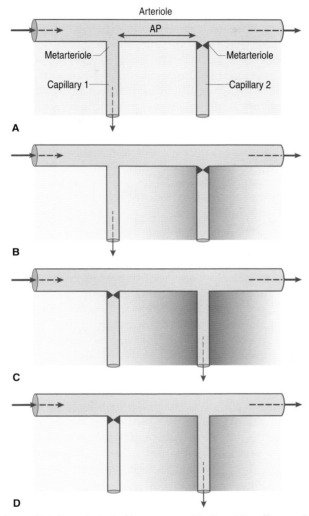

**Figure 6.3** Part of a nutritional vascular bed, with two metarterioles branching off an arteriole and each giving rise to a capillary. (A) The interstitial fluid throughout the region initially contains an even, low concentration of metabolites (shading). With this degree of metabolic dilation of the metarteriolar smooth muscle the absolute input pressure to metarteriole 2 is less than its critical closing pressure, so capillary 2 is not perfused. (B) As a consequence, the local metabolite concentration rises, while metabolites are progressively washed out from the interstitium around capillary 1. (C) When local metabolite concentrations change sufficiently, critical closing pressure in metarteriole 2 becomes less than the input pressure and capillary 2 opens, while metarteriole 1 shuts as its critical closing pressure exceeds the input pressure. (D) As a result, local metabolites begin to accumulate around capillary 1 and are washed out from the area around capillary 2, beginning the sequence again.

upstream capillary is perfused while the more distal capillary has no flow (Fig 6.3A). This will progressively wash metabolites out of the interstitium around the perfused capillary and allow metabolite accumulation around the non-perfused capillary (Fig. 6.3B). In parallel, the relaxant effect of the metabolites will change so that CCP of the perfused metarteriole rises and that of the non-perfused vessel falls. Eventually, CCP in the non-perfused vessel falls below the perfusion pressure so that flow is re-established, while CCP in the perfused vessel will rise above its perfusion pressure and so that metarteriole will shut (Fig. 6.3C–D).

This intermittency of local perfusion takes place typically with a cycle time of 10–30 s, depending on the absolute perfusion pressure and the absolute tissue metabolic rate. Consequently, only around 30% of a resting skeletal muscle is perfused at any one time. Only when metabolic rate rises so far that CCP in all the metarterioles falls below arteriolar perfusion pressure will the entire capillary bed of the tissue be perfused and only under those circumstances of full capillary recruitment can we assume with accuracy that there is a near-linear relationship between blood flow and delivery of blood-borne solutes to specific regions of the tissue. In some vascular beds, however, this may still not mean that there is a proportionate relationship between perfusion pressure and organ blood flow, due to the presence of autoregulation.

It can be envisaged that metarteriolar muscle tone may be subject to tonic dilator influence of EDRFs as well as that of extravascular metabolites. Under these circumstances, EDRFs would accumulate in vessels without blood flow and be depleted by washout in vessels with flow, with the same end result of fluctuating critical closing pressure as has been discussed above. It is unknown whether endothelial factors do contribute significantly to vasomotion, but the relatively long duration of the oscillations could be argued as being more consistent with varying metabolite build-up than with varying EDRF clearance.

It is worth remembering that when vascular smooth muscle is maximally relaxed, CCP approaches zero. Thus, during exercise, the metarterioles in active skeletal muscles will all be open despite the presence of sympathetic vasoconstriction in the arteriolar bed further upstream. As is discussed in Chapter 8 (p. 94), this allows a substantial increase in nutritional muscle perfusion without the need for abolition of local sympathetic tone.

## FUNCTIONAL HYPERAEMIA DURING EXERCISE

### Skeletal muscle circulation

During exercise, nutritional blood flow through the active skeletal muscles rises by 10–20-fold from its resting value of 2–5 ml/min/100 g. This functional hyperaemia reaches a plateau within 2 s of muscle contraction beginning and is maintained throughout the exercise. Although a number of dilator metabolites are known to be produced within contracting muscles, including protons, adenine breakdown products and lactate, none of these substances alone appears to be the primary mediator of the functional hyperaemia, since in no case does the timecourse and concentration profile of metabolite appearance in the interstitium parallel exactly the timecourse and magnitude of hyperaemia (Clifford & Hellsten 2004).

It is likely, therefore, that the full hyperaemic effect represents contributions from a number of metabolites, at least partly through their combined effect on interstitial osmolality. Not even this, however, can explain the rapidity with which blood flow rises at the start of exercise, since no significant release of metabolites has been detected over the first few seconds of contraction. This early phase of hyperaemia seems to be due entirely to release of potassium ions associated with each muscle action potential. Such an effect may seem counter-intuitive since increased extracellular potassium is traditionally thought of as causing depolarization and activation of muscle cells. At concentrations up to around four times the normal extracellular level of 4 mMol; however, potassium selectively relaxes vascular muscle cells by activating a population of inwardly rectifying ($K_{IR}$) channels that cause hyperpolarization.

Other sets of factors also help bring about hyperaemia in exercising muscle, although it is not possible to estimate how much each contribute to blood flow in different patterns of exercise. One is circulating adrenaline (epinephrine), which may activate dilator β-adrenoceptors on the arteriolar muscle, although the effect of this is limited by the presence also of α-adrenoceptors (see Chapter 7, p. 85). As well, contraction leads to release from muscle cells of NO and PGs, more prominently in oxidative than in glycolytic fibres. Thirdly, there is a direct relaxant effect on vascular smooth muscle of the increased tissue temperature associated with increased metabolism (McMeeken & Bell 1990).

These effects on arteriolar tone are supplemented by dilation of the vessels immediately upstream, including the most distal conducting arteries. Despite the arterioles contributing most to regional vascular resistance, arterial dilation reduces regional resistance somewhat and so enhances absolute tissue perfusion. The dilation of conducting arteries appears to involve retrograde propagation of a relaxing signal from the arteriolar level by direct coupling between cells in the vessel wall. The mechanisms underlying this *conducted* (or *propagated*) *dilation* are not well-defined, but may involve endothelial NO and ATP-sensitive potassium channel activation (Takano et al 2005). Finally, the increased blood flow due to all these factors will increase endothelial shear stress in the conduit arteries supplying the active muscles, producing local release of NO and PGs, and reducing overall regional vascular resistance further.

Here is our flow chart (Fig. 6.4) of the matrix of responses to acute exercise, updated to include the effects of these local vasodilator processes.

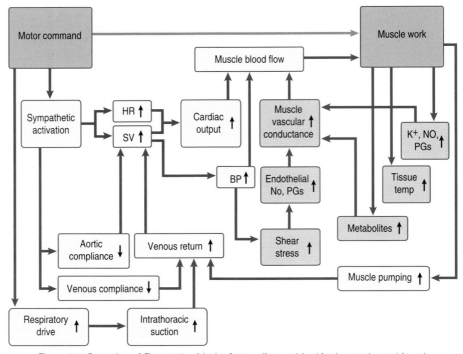

**Figure 6.4** Expansion of Figure 4.2, with the factors discussed in this chapter denoted in red.

## Coronary circulation

Local processes are involved also in the hyperaemic effects of exercise on perfusion of the coronary and cutaneous circulations. The coronary circulation is of course in a state of functional hyperaemia even under non-exercising conditions, reflecting the fact that cardiac muscle is continually active. This means that there is no spare capillary capacity to be drawn on when cardiac workload is increased as evidenced by the fact that oxygen extraction in the coronary capillary bed is always around 60%. By contrast, extraction of oxygen in tissues such as skeletal muscle while at rest, where only a fraction of the capillary bed is perfused at any moment (see Vasomotion, above), is around 30–40%. Under these circumstances, coronary blood flow cannot rise during exercise to the same extent as that in skeletal muscle, the absolute change being proportional to the rise in cardiac output; that is, reaching a ceiling of four to fivefold the resting value in an untrained subject.

β-adrenoceptor activation contributes around 25% of this hyperaemia, the effect being more profound than in skeletal muscle because coronary smooth muscle has a higher ratio of β- to α-adrenoceptors. The magnitude of this sympathetic effect alone is probably sufficient to account for the initial rapid rise in coronary perfusion that is needed to maintain aerobic metabolism over the first few seconds of exercise. The remaining, dominant fraction of the sustained flow increase is presumably mediated primarily by myocardial metabolites and endothelial factors, as in skeletal muscle. However, again as with skeletal muscle, it is clear that no one identified factor is responsible (Tune et al 2004). Assuming that the full response involves cooperative effects of a range of mediators is simpler than postulating that a potent, as-yet undiscovered dilator process exists.

## Skin circulation

Onset of heat-loss processes during sustained exercise involves withdrawal of sympathetic vasomotor drive to the resistance vessels of the skin and a substantial rise in cutaneous blood flow. This passive neural mechanism, however, accounts only for around 50% of the level to which skin blood flow rises during intensive exercise. The remainder of the cutaneous hyperaemic response is secondary to activation of eccrine sweat glands. In these and in other exocrine glands, the secretory process results in liberation of short-chain peptides of the kinin group (bradykinin and kallidin) into the gland interstitium. Kinins are potent vasodilators that act at least partly by stimulating release of endothelial dilator factors (Quyumi & Ozkor 2006). As well as being vasodilators, kinins increase capillary permeability and this facilitates movement of water and electrolytes out of the plasma into the secretory cells.

## Splanchnic circulation

During digestion, blood flow to the digestive tract rises around 10-fold. This profound functional hyperaemia is likely due in part to the effects of local metabolites and endothelial factors, as with cardiac and skeletal muscle. There are, nonetheless, significant contributions also from two other local factors. Like the sweat glands, the gastric, intestinal and pancreatic exocrine glands release kinins in association with the formation of their various secretory products. In addition, the peptide hormones gastrin, secretin, cholecystokinin and vasoactive intestinal peptide all have dilator actions as well as their primary regulatory functions on gut secretion and motility. The overall consequence of this spectrum of metabolism-linked hyperaemic factors is that the vasoconstrictor effect of sympathetic neural activation becomes severely limited. Therefore, when digestion is in progress, the digestive tract circulation ceases to be an effective site of high peripheral resistance to balance the low resistance in exercising muscle. As a result, exercise may be associated with reduced blood pressure, resulting in muscle cramps due to inadequate perfusion and, potentially, loss of consciousness due to inadequate cerebral perfusion.

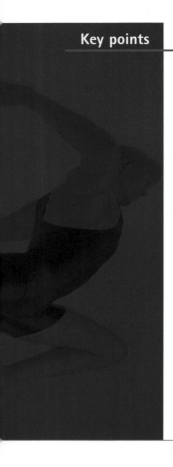

## Key points

The precapillary resistance vessels are subject to substantial local influences that modulate their responsiveness to sympathetic nervous activation.

The most complex of these influences is endothelial dilator factors.

Endothelial dilator capacity is usually assessed from the local dilation following brief arterial occlusion. This reactive hyperaemia occurs in both conduit and microcirculatory arterial vessels, but the underlying processes differ and it is not clear which site provides the best assessment of physiological endothelial function.

Dilator actions of extracellular tissue metabolites and the constrictor effects of increased smooth muscle membrane tension are also important in local control of vascular resistance.

Collectively, these local factors act to maintain local nutritional perfusion at a level appropriate to the metabolic demand of the tissue in the face of alterations in perfusion pressure.

During aerobic exercise, the rapid initial hyperaemia in skeletal muscle involves efflux of potassium ion from the muscle cells.

The maintained elevation of muscle blood flow is due to the combined dilator effects of a number of local factors, including metabolites and other substances released from the active muscle cells, endothelial mediators and elevated temperature.

## References

Barry MA 2003 Effects of smoking and ageing on cardiovascular function. PhD thesis, University of Dublin.

Clifford PS, Hellsten Y 2004 Vasodilatory mechanisms in contracting skeletal muscle. Journal of Applied Physiology 97: 393–403.

Dora KA 2005 Does arterial myogenic tone determine blood flow in vivo? American Journal of Physiology 289: H1323–H1325.

Hansell J, Hemareh L, Agewall S, Norman M 2004 Non-invasive assessment of endothelial function – relation between vasodilatory responses in skin microcirculation and brachial artery. Clinical Physiology and Functional Imaging 24: 317–322.

McMeeken JM, Bell C 1990 Microwave irradiation of the human forearm and hand. Physiotherapy, Theory & Practice 6: 171–176.

O'Sullivan SE 2003 The effects of exercise training on markers of endothelial function in young healthy men. International Journal of Sports Medicine 24: 404–409.

Quayle JM, Turner MR, Burrell HE, Kamishima T 2006 Effects of hypoxia, anoxia, and metabolic inhibitors on KATP channels in rat femoral artery myocytes. American Journal of the Heart, Circulation and Physiology 291: H71–H80.

Quyyumi AA, Ozkor M 2006 Vasodilation by hyperpolarization: beyond NO. Hypertension 48: 1023–1025.

Rassaf T, Heiss C, Hendgen-Cotta U et al 2006 Plasma nitrite reserve and endothelial function in the human forearm circulation. Free Radical Biology and Medicine 41: 295–301.

Takano H, Dora KA, Garland CJ 2005 Spreading vasodilatation in resistance arteries. Journal of Smooth Muscle Research 41: 303–311.

Tune JD, Gorman MW, Feigl EO 2004 Matching coronary blood flow to myocardial oxygen consumption. Journal of Applied Physiology 97: 404–415.

## Questions for revision

- List the identities and sources of chemical factors that have been implicated in local regulation of blood flow.

- What is reactive hyperaemia and how can it be measured?

- Describe the process involved in the myogenic response and indicate how this phenomenon may function to regulate regional blood flow.

- Define autoregulation and discuss how it is achieved.

- Write notes on the phenomenon of vasomotion.

- During exercise, blood flow to the active skeletal muscles rises dramatically. Discuss the factors that underlie this hyperaemia.

## Chapter 7

# Central nervous system control of cardiovascular function

### CHAPTER CONTENTS

## After reading this chapter, you should:

- understand the basic patterns of brain control over sympathetic cardiovascular pathways
- be able to predict how cerebral arousal and exercise affect blood pressure and regional blood flows
- appreciate the different effects of dynamic and resistive exercise on these parameters

The brain exerts powerful effects on cardiovascular behaviour, predominantly by altering sympathetic motor drive to the heart and to vascular smooth muscle. While you may read about sympathetic activation specifically in relation to cardiac function or arteriolar resistance or venous capacitance, depending on the topic being discussed, the truth is that centrally mediated sympathetic activation almost always involves increased drive to both heart and blood vessels and in non-selective increases in vasomotor drive to arteries and veins. Therefore, heart rate and blood pressure usually change in parallel. This parallelism is convenient because it means that changes in any of these parameters can be used as an (approximate) index of sympathetic activation. In practice, the parameter used routinely is the change in heart rate, because

ECGs can be recorded continually in moving subjects so much more easily than blood pressure.

## ORGANIZATION OF CENTRAL CARDIOVASCULAR CONTROL

Although sympathetic outflow to the cardiovascular system can be affected by pathways arising in many areas of the brain, there are for our purposes three primary sources of this activation (Fig. 7.1). The first is the cardiovascular control centre lying in the medulla of the hindbrain, which is the final common pathway for all descending sympathetic information. This hindbrain centre receives reflex inputs directly from peripheral sensory nerves, but also receives descending inputs from two areas of the forebrain. The most important of these are the limbic system, which includes the hypothalamus and several neighbouring nuclei, mediates emotional arousal and determines levels of consciousness, and the motor cortex from which all instructions for muscle movement must originate.

Neuroscientists are still unravelling the specific neural connections and neurotransmitters involved in mediation of hindbrain regulation of the cardiovascular system. However, we can regard the cardiovascular control centre as consisting of two sets of tonically active descending neurons, one producing continual activation of the sympathetic outflows to heart and blood vessels and one producing continual inhibition of heart rate via the vagus (Fig. 7.2). As a result of this ongoing activity, there is usually some degree of vasoconstrictor tone in both arterial and venous vessels, while the heart rate at rest reflects the algebraic sum of inputs to the sinoatrial node of both sympathetic and vagal activity.

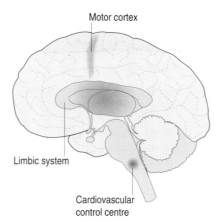

Motor cortex

Limbic system

Cardiovascular
control centre

**Figure 7.1** Diagrammatic saggital view of the brain, showing the locations of the hindbrain cardiovascular control centre and the two most powerful forebrain activators of hindbrain sympathetic drive; the limbic system and the motor cortex.

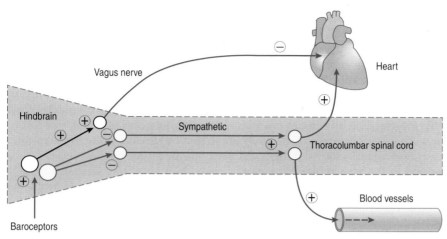

**Figure 7.2** A simplified version of the neural circuitry of the hindbrain cardiovascular control centre and its baroreceptor inputs. Primary sensory inputs from baroreceptive neurons communicate via a series of interneurons as shown, to activate vagal outflow and to inhibit sympathetic outflow. Excitatory and inhibitory synaptic inputs are indicated by (+) and (−).

# LOW–PRESSURE AND HIGH–PRESSURE BAROREFLEXES

## Baroreflex effects on sympathetic cardiovascular control

The moment-to-moment regulation of blood pressure is via reflexes that operate through inputs to the hindbrain centre from mechanosensitive sensory axons monitoring pressure in the aorta and the carotid arteries (*high-pressure baroreceptors*) and in the atria (*low-pressure baroreceptors*). In all cases, increased distension results in increased sensory firing and the sensory neurons inhibit activity of the hindbrain centre sympathetic neurons. In consequence, either increased blood pressure or increased central blood volume will reduce peripheral resistance, while falls in blood pressure or central blood volume have the opposite effects.

With high pressure baroreflexes, parallel changes in cardiac and vascular sympathetic drive are seen, so that a reflex fall in peripheral resistance is accompanied by bradycardia. Although for ease of measurement the magnitude of baroreflex responses is usually assessed in terms of heart rate changes, it should be remembered that the end-point of the reflex is blood pressure regulation and that adjustment of peripheral resistance rather than heart rate is the dominant factor in achieving this.

Low-pressure baroreflexes have a distinct pattern of cardiac and vascular responses, with reflex falls in peripheral resistance caused by increased atrial filling being usually accompanied by tachycardia. However, increases in atrial volume that raise stroke volume will also induce an arterial baroreflex and bradycardia. This means that heart rate changes may be an uncertain index of baroreflex activity since their magnitude will vary depending on the algebraic sum of low-pressure and high-pressure receptor inputs.

Although the arterial and atrial pressure-sensitive sensory axons are commonly referred to as baroreceptors, they are in fact simple stretch receptors that react to vessel wall distortion rather than to the transmural pressure itself. For this reason, arterial baroreceptors cannot detect intravascular pressures below around 40 mmHg because there is insufficient wall stretch. Further, increased stiffness of the arterial wall by smooth muscle contraction, loss of elastic tissue or infiltration with inorganic precipitates such as calcium can greatly dampen recognition of intravascular pressure changes. As mechanoreceptors, the baroreceptors also respond to the rate of distortion as well as to its magnitude, so that during the arterial pulse wave they fire more during the rising phase than at equivalent absolute pressure levels during the falling phase.

Because the purpose of the baroreflex is to achieve restoration of arterial or atrial pressure to its operating point as efficiently as possible, it is not surprising that baroreflex activation involves the regulation of vasoconstrictor tone in large vascular beds that can contribute most to total peripheral resistance – skeletal muscle, digestive tract and kidneys. All three of these beds are equally involved in arterial baroreflex responses. Atrial baroreflexes appear to have a preferential effect on renal resistance, reflecting their involvement in blood volume regulation.

The cutaneous circulation, which is the other large vascular bed in the body, is recruited to only a small extent by baroreflex adjustments, allowing it to be reserved entirely for thermoregulatory regulation. Notwithstanding, thermoregulatory and baroreflex demands can interact, since the vascular response to body heating involves withdrawal of sympathetic vasomotor tone not only from the cutaneous arterioles, but also from both small and large superficial veins in the limbs. The consequent increase in venous volume reduces circulating blood volume and so reduces the efficiency with which baroreflex adjustments are able to compensate for postural change.

## Baroreflex effects on hormonal cardiovascular control

The immediate neural compensations to altered blood pressure or blood volume are supplemented by concomitant changes in hormone release that provide longer-term reinforcement of the response. If blood pressure or atrial pressure falls, increased sympathetic discharge to the kidney not only increases renal vascular resistance, but also activates release of the enzyme renin from juxtaglomerular cells in the afferent arteriolar wall. Released renin cleaves the octapeptide angiotensin I from the circulating liver derived precursor angiotensinogen, and the angiotensin I is converted to angiotensin II by angiotensin-converting enzyme (ACE) in the pulmonary endothelium. Angiotensin II is a potent vasoconstrictor agent. It also stimulates release of aldosterone from the adrenal cortex, so retarding renal excretion of sodium and increasing blood volume.

Activation of low-pressure baroreceptors by atrial distension sends inhibitory inputs to the hypothalamus that depress release of vasopressin (antidiuretic hormone, ADH) from the posterior pituitary gland. As a result, less water is reabsorbed from the renal collecting ducts and plasma volume is reduced. Conversely, reduced atrial baroreceptor activity due to lower atrial pressure will increase vasopressin release, retaining water and elevating plasma volume.

## Baroreflexes and 'resting' cardiovascular status

In most experiments concerned with human cardiovascular responses, it is essential to obtain baseline values for heart rate and blood pressure at rest. Standardization of posture is an important factor here, since upright posture inevitably results in heightened sympathetic drive. This is due to baroreflex recognition of reduced venous return because of venous pooling in the legs and splanchnic area. Ideally, baseline data should be obtained with subjects supine so as to ensure complete abolition of gravitational forces on the venous system. However, in practical terms this is often difficult to reconcile with the other requirements of the experiment – access to equipment, comfort of the subject while viewing a display screen, etc. – and the majority of studies use the seated position as a realistic compromise.

Whichever posture is adopted, the experimenter must be aware that, although the baroreflex responds rapidly to postural change, at least several minutes are needed for the situation to stabilize. This is due in part to the timecourse of removal of catecholamines from the bloodstream and partly to the relatively slow rebalancing of fluid between bloodstream and interstitium in the lower legs after intracapillary pressure falls. Pre-measurement equilibration times are routinely around 10 min. This ignores the fact that circulating angiotensin and vasopressin may take 15–30 min to stabilize, but these hormones contribute relatively little to total peripheral resistance changes with posture unless the subject has been subjected to previous stress, such as dehydration, that elevate angiotensin and vasopressin secretion.

## AROUSAL AND SYMPATHETIC CARDIOVASCULAR CONTROL: THE LIMBIC SYSTEM

The resting level of cardiovascular sympathetic drive is reduced when the level of cerebral arousal falls (for example, during sleep) and rises with heightened arousal, such as occurs during conversation or performing a mental task. The correlation of absolute heart rate and blood pressure with cerebral activation means that, in order to measure true 'resting' cardiovascular values, subjects should sit quietly and talk as little as possible for at least 10 min before measurements are commenced. Even so, it is often found that the additional arousal induced by measurement causes a transient increase in sympathetic activity; for this reason it is usual to record continuous data for at least 2–3 min and take at least three sets of intermittent data.

When cerebral arousal involves an emotional component – for instance, fright or anxiety – then the degree of sympathetic activation and the pressor response are greater. Emotionally oriented arousal often also produces an additional component of the response; an increase in limb muscle blood flow that is due to active vasodilation of the muscle arteriolar bed. The potential functional significance of this response has been the subject of extensive investigation over more than 50 years, without definitive resolution. Studies in cats and dogs have shown that the dilation is mediated by activation of sympathetic cholinergic vasodilator nerves. These nerves are activated from areas of the limbic system that also cause the behavioural changes known as the 'flight and fight' or 'defence' reaction, leading to the proposal that they might provide instantaneous high muscle blood flow at the commencement of exercise associated with escape or aggression.

In man, emotionally oriented arousal can cause profound forearm muscle vasodilation and this response has been shown in some studies to be dependent on sympathetic nerve integrity and abolished by acetylcholine antagonists, such as atropine. Other studies, by contrast, have found the response to be independent of local sympathetic innervation and sensitive to β-adrenoreceptor antagonists or inhibitors of nitric oxide, but not to atropine. Other studies again report that emotional stimuli evoke only generalized vasoconstriction. The basis of arousal-linked muscle dilatation in man is, therefore, still uncertain, except in so far that it is clearly not as straightforward as in some other species (Joyner & Dietz 2003). More importantly, it remains unknown whether such a response would confer any physiological advantage to muscle perfusion on initiation of exercise over and above that provided by local dilator factors released from the contracting muscle cells (see Chapter 6, p. 64). If there were a functional role, then it might be postulated to be most likely of significance for short, repetitive, sub-tetanic activity that does not release sufficient local factors from the muscle cells to induce optimal dilatation. So, for example, a role in playing musical instruments is possible. However, a role in whole-body exercise seems unlikely, although the rise in blood pressure induced by limbic arousal may itself provide some instantaneous benefit for muscle perfusion over the first few seconds of an anticipated exercise.

## SYMPATHETIC CARDIOVASCULAR CONTROL DURING EXERCISE

### Pressor effect of exercise

Once exercise commences, blood pressure rises rapidly and proportionately to the intensity of activity, regardless of whether or not the activity is anticipated. This pressor response involves a number of sympathetic effector pathways from the hindbrain cardiovascular centre together with release of adrenaline (*epinephrine*) from the adrenal medulla, causing generalized vasoconstriction of smooth muscle in both venous and arterial vessels. Decreased venous reservoir function increases venous return and stroke volume, decreased aortic compliance increases systolic blood pressure (SBP) and arteriolar constriction increases diastolic blood pressure (DBP).

#### Sites of peripheral resistance increase

Increased activity of arteriolar constrictor nerves during exercise appears to be generalized across all major regional beds except the brain. In terms of absolute resistance changes, the effects on circulations to the splanchnic region and the kidneys are most pronounced, with blood flows to these areas falling by as much as 70–80% during maximal exertion. In the kidneys, sympathetic activation preferentially constricts the efferent arterioles downstream of the glomeruli, so elevating glomerular capillary pressure. This allows relatively efficient filtration to continue despite the low absolute perfusion.

During exercise, absolute blood flow to skeletal and cardiac muscles rises with work intensity, reflecting the increased local metabolic needs and due in the main to a variety of local dilator processes (see Chapter 6, pp. 72–74). The maximum levels of flow achieved reflect the increments in tissue activity that occur, being 10–20-fold for skeletal muscle (from 1 l/min to 10–20 l/min) and around four-fold for the coronary circulation (from 250 ml/min to 1 l/min). However, the sympathetic activation that accompanies exercise is not region-specific, so there is increased vasoconstrictor drive to skeletal muscle and the heart as well as to splanchnic and renal beds. Thus, the maximum nutritional perfusion that can be achieved in these tissues are less than would be predicted on the basis of the dilator stimuli alone.

Several aspects of this interaction between dilator and constrictor processes bear mention. First, the presence of sympathetic vasoconstriction in skeletal muscle contributes to total peripheral resistance during intense dynamic exercise, and appears to be essential in order to allow maintenance of adequate blood pressure. Second, there is evidence that at near-maximum dynamic exercise intensities, muscle oxygenation may become limited by the sympathetic constrictor effect (Mortensen et al 2005). Third, although vasoconstriction limits the blood flow to exercising skeletal muscle to levels substantially lower than would exist if there were unopposed dilatation, nutritional capillary perfusion during exercise is significantly greater than indicated by the fall in muscle vascular resistance. This is because only around 30% of the capillary bed is perfused in resting skeletal muscle (see Chapter 6, p. 72). Recruitment of the remainder of the capillary bed by metabolite-induced reduction of metarteriolar critical closing pressure provides a threefold elevation in tissue perfusion before there is any requirement for reduced arteriolar resistance.

There is evidence that in the coronary circulation also, sympathetic activation has less effect on nutritional perfusion than is suggested by the absolute effect on regional resistance. This is due to the fact that, in the coronary vasculature, the α-adrenoreceptors are localized primarily to the largest arterioles and small arteries. The constrictor effect of sympathetic activation on these larger vessels stiffens them and actually increases flow to the deeper regions of myocardium, presumably because it reduces external compression during cardiac contraction (Tune et al 2004).

Finally, it is worth noting that whatever the degree of generalized sympathetic activation, the absolute effect on vascular resistance is greater in splanchnic and renal beds than in skeletal muscle and coronary circulations, because small arterioles in the latter two beds contain dilator β-adrenoreceptors as well as α-adrenoreceptors, while those in splanchnic and renal beds are devoid of β-adrenoreceptors.

## Origin of signals for sympathetic activation

All forms of exercise depend on descending information from the upper motor neurons of motor cortex to the lower motor neurons controlling muscle contraction. The upper motor neurons also send excitatory inputs to the cardiovascular control centre, so that peripheral vasoconstriction, tachycardia and increased cardiac contraction occur proportionately to both the amount of musculature activated and the intensity of activation. This input to cardiovascular regulation from the motor cortex is known as *central command*. Although it has traditionally been viewed as originating solely from the cortex, recent studies using imaging and electrophysiological recording indicate that areas of the limbic system are also involved (Green et al 2007).

Two additional signals provide additional input to the cardiovascular control centre. Mechanoreceptors in the limb joints and in the limb musculature give information on the amount and speed of muscle contraction. As well, chemoreceptors within the muscle interstitium detect accumulation of metabolites. Both these signals have the capacity to enhance the sympatho-excitatory effect of central command during any modality of exercise, but limb mechanoreceptors will be activated predominantly during dynamic exercise, while chemoreceptors are activated far more during static exercise when muscle perfusion is minimized by external compression. Evidence from studies of static exercise indicates also that the effect of chemoreceptor activation (the so-called *metaboreflex*) is preferentially on vasoconstrictor function, with relatively little effect on cardiac function.

Figure 7.3 adds the factors discussed above to our flow chart of the exercise response.

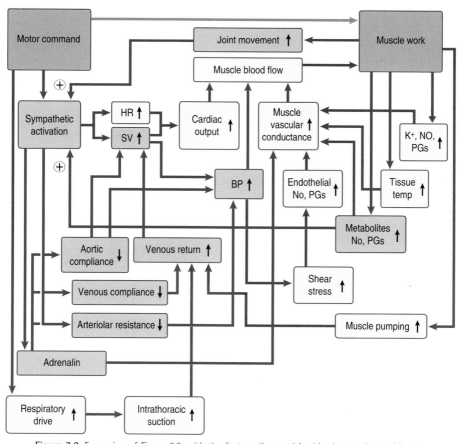

**Figure 7.3** Expansion of Figure 6.3, with the factors discussed in this chapter denoted in red.

## Comparison of dynamic and static exercise

The different contributions from different signals of motor activity, together with the circulatory effects of the exercise itself, result in distinct patterns of pressor and cardioaccelerator responses to dynamic and to static exercise. During dynamic exercise, sympathetic activation is determined primarily by central command, so that maximal tachycardia and blood pressure are achieved only when a large proportion of the whole-body musculature is involved. Under these conditions, heart rate will attain its age-dependent maximum (see Chapter 4, p. 32) and SBP will rise substantially due to the combined effects of tachycardia, increased stroke volume and reduced aortic compliance. DBP is not usually elevated during dynamic exercise because of the large fall in total peripheral resistance. At low-to-moderate workloads, the reduced resistance is balanced by tachycardia and DBP remains unchanged from the resting value (Fig. 7.4A). At high workloads in the upright posture, by contrast, DBP often begins to fall because of the profound reduction in total peripheral resistance caused by maximal muscle vasodilation.

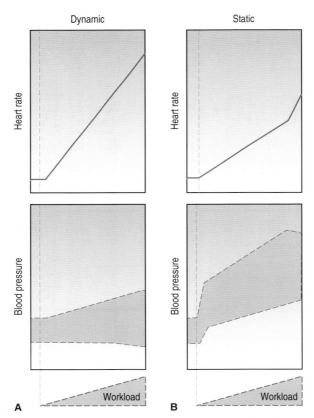

**Figure 7.4** Representative changes in heart rate and blood pressure during increasing intensities of dynamic and static work. Note the very different effects on blood pressure of the two exercise modalities. Note also the inflections in heart rate and blood pressure curves at peak static workloads, due to obstructed venous return.

The picture seen during static exercise is strikingly different (Fig. 7.4B). For one thing, substantial elevation of SBP and heart rate occurs not only with whole-body exercise, but is seen with contraction of quite small muscle groups, such as those controlling handgrip. This is due in a large part to metaboreflex input, secondary to mechanical compression of the muscle vascular supply. In addition, since peripheral resistance does not fall during static exercise, but actually rises due to compression of the muscle vasculature, DBP rises with workload. Finally, increased intra-abdominal and intra-thoracic pressures during whole-body static activity progressively reduce venous return and stroke volume, leading to blood pressure actually falling slightly at peak workload.

Resistance exercises, such as rowing and weight-lifting, have some characteristics of both dynamic and static activities, and, not surprisingly, the circulatory responses also have a mixed pattern, the details of which vary widely with the intensity and duration of exercise. Thus, weight-training with low loads and many repetitions may have little more effect than purely dynamic exercise on blood pressure, whereas pressing a single 100% repetition-maximum load can raise SBP to the order of 300 mmHg – far more than is ever seen during dynamic activity.

## Comparison of upper–body and lower–body exercise

Selective upper-body exercise constitutes the basis of fitness training for patients with limited mobility or spinal cord injury. The heart rate achieved at maximum workload is similar to that seen with whole-body exercise, but the absolute achievable workload and the maximum cardiac output are lower because of the smaller muscle mass involved. In addition, heart rate increments are greater for given increments of work than when whole-body exercise takes place, because the absence of muscle pumping in the legs reduces the venous pressure gradient and limits ventricular filling (see Chapter 3, p. 22).

Upper-body exercise is also characterized by greater elevation of blood pressure than is whole-body or selective lower-body activity. Most strikingly, there is a rise in DBP as well as in SBP. This is due primarily to the fact that the sympathetic vasoconstriction of lower limb musculature is not attenuated by functional vasodilation in the same muscles, so total peripheral resistance is higher. A smaller contribution may come from metaboreflex activation, since most upper-body ergometers require the subject to grip the winding cranks and this introduces a degree of static exercise.

## BAROREFLEX RESETTING IN EXERCISE

It is clear from the preceding discussion that exercise is associated with maintenance of blood pressure at levels significantly higher than that during rest. This pressure elevation serves two purposes. First, it optimizes nutritional perfusion of the various organ systems in the face of increased regional vasoconstrictor tone. Second, suddenly stopping exercise would immediately stop muscle pumping in the legs, causing a fall in venous return and cardiac output that might prejudice cerebral perfusion in the upright posture. The pre-existence of elevated sympathetic vasoconstriction makes this less likely.

In order to achieve a sustained blood pressure elevation, it is necessary for there to be resetting of the baroreflexes that would otherwise tend to counteract the exercise-induced sympathetic activation. In terms of high-pressure baroreceptor function, this is achieved by upward adjustment of the baroreflex operating point, so that blood pressure is regulated around a value greater than at rest. The extent of the upwards shift in operating point is dependent on exercise intensity and presumably is mediated at least mainly by inputs to the baroreflex pathway of messages from central command. It is not known whether the function of low-pressure baroreflexes is also affected by exercise.

## POST–EXERCISE HYPOTENSION

Cessation of exercise is necessarily associated with cessation of the central command for sympathetic activation. This could, in theory, lead to a temporary situation in which widespread vasodilation in skeletal muscle due to residual interstitial metabolites, unopposed by sympathetic vasoconstriction in both muscle and splanchnic beds, would cause a precipitous fall in blood pressure. The fact that this does not normally occur even after intense exercise may reflect the persistence of baroreflex resetting for a period after termination of activity.

Nonetheless, it has been found in a number of studies that blood pressure sometimes falls after dynamic exercise to values slightly below those recorded pre-exercise, over a period of 10–20 min, and that this post-exercise hypotension may be maintained for at least several hours; in some studies up to almost a day. The mechanisms underlying post-exercise hypotension are not well defined, except in as far as (by definition) it must involve some downwards resetting of baroreflex function. Studies in which sympathetic activity has been monitored show reduced vasomotor drive, but some other studies suggest a primary effect on neural control of cardiac function. Evidence from animals, in which a similar hypotensive response is seen, indicate that it involves effects on the baroreflex pathway of opioids released within the hindbrain during exercise.

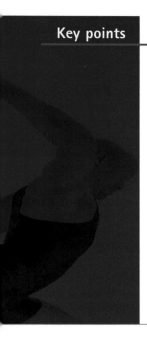

## Key points

Autonomic control of blood pressure and heart rate originates from the cardiovascular control centre of the hindbrain.

Limbic system activation of the hindbrain centre has the consequence that blood pressure and heart rate rise with increased arousal, regardless of the cause.

Motor cortical activation of the hindbrain centre provides automatic coupling of blood pressure and heart rate increments to the amount of muscle work being performed.

In addition, sympathetic drive is further activated during exercise by sensory inputs that monitor the extent of limb movement and the accumulation of metabolites in muscle interstitium.

The maintenance of the changes relies on upward resetting of the baroreceptor operating point.

Cessation of exercise may be followed by a prolonged period of reduced sympathetic vasoconstrictor tone and hypotension.

## References

Green AL, Wang S, Purvis et al 2007 Identifying cardiorespiratory neurocircuitry involved in central command during exercise in humans. Journal of Physiology 578: 605–612.

Joyner MJ, Dietz NM 2003 Sympathetic vasodilation in human muscle. Acta Physiologica Scandinavica 177: 329–336.

Mortensen SP, Dawson EA, Yoshiga CC et al 2005 Limitations to systemic and locomotor limb muscle oxygen delivery and uptake during maximal exercise in humans. Journal of Physiology 566: 273–285.

Tune JD, Gorman MW, Feigl EO 2004 Matching coronary blood flow to myocardial oxygen consumption. Journal of Applied Physiology 97: 404–415.

## Further reading

Biaggioni I 2007 Autonomic/metabolic interactions modulating the exercise pressor reflex: the purinergic hypothesis. Journal of Physiology 578: 5–6.

Rezk CC, Marrache RCB, Tinucci T, Mion D Jr, Forjaz CLM 2006 Post-resistance exercise hypotension, hemodynamics, and heart rate variability: influence of exercise intensity. European Journal of Applied Physiology 98: 105–112.

Rowell LB 2004 Ideas about control of skeletal and cardiac muscle blood flow (1876–2003): cycles of revision and new vision. Journal of Applied Physiology 97: 384–392.

### Questions for revision

- Discuss the baroreflex control of blood pressure.

- Describe the neural circuitry involved in hindbrain control of cardiovascular function.

- What is 'central command'?
- What factors cause blood pressure elevation during resistive exercise?
- Explain the differences between circulatory responses to exercise using an arm cranker and a cycle ergometer.

# Chapter 8

# Pulmonary circulation

## CHAPTER CONTENTS

## After reading this chapter, you should:

- understand the advantages and disadvantages of the low perfusion pressure gradient through the pulmonary circulation
- know the mechanisms by which ventilation and perfusion are matched during exercise
- understand the changes in heart and pulmonary perfusion that accompany birth
- appreciate the implications for pulmonary vascular function of some common congenital cardiovascular defects

The pulmonary circulation is contained wholly within the thorax. It is, therefore, much shorter than most regional beds of the systemic circulation. As well, all segments of the pulmonary vessels are slightly larger in radius than the corresponding segments of the systemic vasculature. The net result of these two factors is that the pulmonary circulation exerts a resistance to flow only around 15% of that in the systemic circuit. Hence it requires a correspondingly far lower pressure gradient in order to move the same cardiac output. At rest, pulmonary arterial pressure is typically 25/8 mmHg, giving a mean arterial pressure of the order of 14 mmHg, and mean pulmonary capillary pressure is 7–8 mmHg rather than the 25–30 mmHg seen in systemic vascular beds.

## FUNCTIONAL CONSEQUENCES OF LOW PULMONARY BLOOD PRESSURE

### Gas diffusion

In systemic capillaries the balance between oncotic and hydrostatic pressures mean that small increases in hydrostatic pressure caused, for example, by reduced arteriolar resistance will result in significant movement of plasma water into the interstitium. When a large tissue mass, such as skeletal muscle, is involved, this movement will cause a substantial reduction of plasma volume (see Chapter 9, p. 112), but the increased interstitial volume does not prejudice diffusion of solutes between cells and bloodstream because the intercellular connective tissue minimizes tissue expansion. In the lung, by contrast, there is little supporting tissue. If water moves into the interstitial space separating the pulmonary capillaries from the alveoli, it pushes these two structures further apart and increases the distance over which gases must diffuse between air and plasma.

The speed of this diffusional process decreases very rapidly with increased distance, so efficient lung function depends on minimizing the interstitial space by keeping it free of extra water. A pulmonary capillary hydrostatic pressure of 7–8 mmHg is three times less than plasma oncotic pressure. Therefore, there is normally quite a large net inward osmotic gradient to maintain this situation. If, however, capillary pressure rises to levels similar to those in systemic capillaries, then interstitial water starts to accumulate (*pulmonary oedema*) and gas exchange may become compromised.

This situation results commonly from damage to the mitral valve that separates left atrium and ventricle. Either valvular stenosis or incompetence will elevate left atrial pressure and this will cause a proportionate change in capillary pressure, which may rise as high as 40–50 mmHg with severe valve damage. Paradoxically, patients in whom chronic valve damage has led to a progressive, slow rise in left atrial pressure often have far less pulmonary oedema than would be expected from the absolute pressure changes. This seems to be because, under these circumstances, the lymphatic system within the lung becomes more efficient in recycling fluid from the interstitial spaces.

The practising exercise physiologist is most likely to encounter pulmonary oedema as a consequence of high altitude, since it occurs in many healthy individuals who ascend to heights greater than 3000 m, well below the altitude of many ski resorts and permanent settlements. We will return to examine the reasons for this response to altitude in Chapter 12 (p. 151).

# Right ventricular function

Left ventricular perfusion occurs only during diastole because during systole the left coronary vessels are compressed by the surrounding cardiac muscle (see Chapter 2, p. 6). By contrast, since right ventricular pressure does not normally rise above 25 mmHg, the coronary vasculature supplying the right ventricle is not compressed at any stage of the cardiac cycle and coronary flow is continuous. The increased efficiency of coronary oxygen delivery is reflected in a lower density of coronary blood vessels in the right heart. However, this design feature has potentially disadvantageous results if left atrial pressure becomes chronically elevated and right ventricular pressure rises in response to this higher afterload.

Under these circumstances, right coronary perfusion during systole becomes progressively reduced and the metabolic demands of the right-side cardiac muscle cells are less efficiently serviced. Over time, the right ventricle will respond to the high afterload by muscle hypertrophy. This will exaggerate the coronary insufficiency, both by providing greater metabolic demand for oxygen delivery and by producing more coronary compression. As a result, chronic hypoxic damage to the muscle of the right heart, with an inability to increase contraction appropriately in response to increased filling (*right cardiac failure*) is a common long-term effect of elevated pulmonary blood pressure (see Chapter 12, p. 148).

## REGIONAL MATCHING OF VENTILATION AND PERFUSION

## Vertical variations

In a resting, upright individual, dramatic differences in both respiratory ventilation and pulmonary perfusion exist along the vertical axis of the lung. Resting inspiration is due to elevation of the ribs and lowering of the diaphragm, but the shape of the ribcage means that the increase in thoracic volume that occurs becomes progressively more pronounced towards the lung bases. The fact that the lung apices are around 10 cm higher than the heart means that the vessels there are perfused only when pulmonary arterial pressure exceeds this value (10 cm $H_2O$ = 14 mmHg). Thus, there is only intermittent apical perfusion, especially during expiration when intra-thoracic pressure rises and compresses the capillaries. By contrast, the lung bases are gravitationally lower than the heart; therefore, the perfusion pressure for vessels in this region is several mmHg higher than that at heart level and perfusion is correspondingly greater.

Although both ventilation and perfusion rise towards the base of the lungs, the gravitational effect on regional blood flow is rather more powerful than the vertical variation in ventilation, with the result that the ratio of ventilation $\dot{V}$ to perfusion $\dot{Q}$ is around 3 at the apices and around 0.5 at

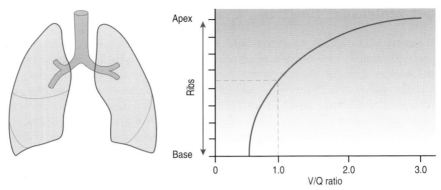

**Figure 8.1** Ventilation/perfusion ($\dot{V}/\dot{Q}$) ratio variation in the vertical lung. At rest, optimal matching ($\dot{V}/\dot{Q}=1.0$) occurs only over a relatively narrow region around the mid-sternal area.

the bases. Exact matching of the two is achieved only over a relatively narrow region of lung corresponding to about the mid-sternal level (Fig. 8.1).

## Effects of intrapulmonary gas tensions

At rest, when tidal volume is around 400–600 ml, the lung does not expand sufficiently during inspiration to allow ventilation of all alveoli. Those at the end of the longest airways with greatest resistance and those that are subjected to the greatest external tissue forces receive little if any fresh air, so that the air within these regions accumulates carbon dioxide and becomes progressively depleted of oxygen. In terms of $\dot{V}/\dot{Q}$ matching, it is clearly more efficient if the pulmonary blood flow bypasses these alveoli and is directed entirely to regions in which the concentration gradients for gas exchange are optimal.

To fulfil this purpose, hypoxia sensors exist within the pulmonary arteriolar walls that monitor the oxygen concentration in adjacent alveoli (the $P_AO_2$). We have seen previously that this receptor type is found in systemic arterioles, where it mediates a hyperpolarizing vasodilator response to hypoxia (Chapter 6, p. 68). In pulmonary arterioles, by contrast, hypoxia receptor activation causes muscle cell depolarization and vasoconstriction. The subcellular mechanisms that transduce this process are still the subject of debate; oxygen-sensitive potassium channels appear to be involved, but evidence exists also for release of some endothelium-derived vasoactive factor (Moudgil et al 2005). The terminal airways also possess receptors that detect locally inefficient ventilation – mainly by recognizing carbon dioxide build-up rather than oxygen depletion – and this dilates the airways and so helps re-oxygenate the under-ventilated alveoli. The interaction of arteriolar receptors for hypoxia and airway receptors for hypercapnia means that the regions of poor perfusion do not remain constant but oscillate in response to the oscillations in regional ventilation.

When hypoxic vasoconstriction affects small regions of the lung during normal air breathing, it helps optimize the efficiency of gas exchange. If, however, one were to breathe air that contained less oxygen than usual, then there would be widespread vasoconstriction and an increase in total pulmonary vascular resistance that would increase right heart workload. We shall look at this situation further when we examine the circulatory effects of high altitude in Chapter 12 (p. 143).

## CHANGES IN PULMONARY EFFICIENCY WITH EXERCISE

Even at peak workloads, pulmonary gas exchange is usually unimpaired and arterial oxygen saturation remains unchanged from rest. One factor in this maintenance of optimal gas exchange is that, with a normal resting cardiac output, equilibrium between alveolar air and plasma is reached about one-third of the way along a typical pulmonary capillary. Thus, full oxygen saturation of blood can be maintained when cardiac output rises around threefold without any additional adjustments being needed. At higher work intensities, additional mechanisms must be employed to maintain gas exchange. These involve increasing the efficiency of matching between perfusion and ventilation.

The increased respiratory drive that automatically accompanies motor cortex activation increases minute ventilation proportionately to exercise intensity. This both expands regions of the lung that are partially collapsed at rest, removing external compression of the microcirculatory vessels, and causes pulmonary arteriolar dilation due to elevation of $P_AO_2$ in these areas.

In addition, the increased depth of breathing results in greater intrathoracic negative pressure during inspiration, which increases right atrial filling, right stroke volume and pulmonary arterial pressure. This produces more efficient perfusion of lung areas that are gravitationally above the heart.   Collectively, these factors transform the variable regional $\dot{V}/\dot{Q}$

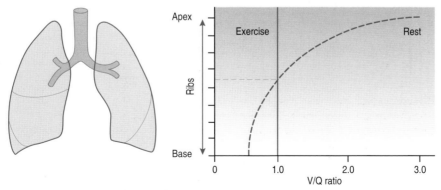

**Figure 8.2** Ventilation/perfusion ratio variation in the vertical lung during intense whole-body exercise. Note that now, by contrast with the situation at rest, there is optimal matching throughout the lung.

relationship to one that is virtually independent of vertical position (Fig. 8.2). In addition, distribution of blood flow over a greater number of pulmonary capillaries reduces the velocity of flow through each of these and so increases the time for oxygen loading.

Figure 8.3 adds the contributions of pulmonary circulation and lungs to our flow chart of the exercise response.

Although the processes outlined above are able in most individuals to preserve optimal uptake of oxygen, even at the highest work intensities, there is one population in whom pulmonary gas exchange does limit work capacity under normoxic conditions. In a proportion of elite athletes with work capacities of the order of 70 ml $O_2$/min/kg, arterial oxygen saturation falls from the normal of 96–97% to as low as around 90% at peak exercise (Stewart & Pickering 2006). It appears that these individuals generate cardiac outputs during exercise which are so high that, even with optimal $\dot{V}/\dot{Q}$

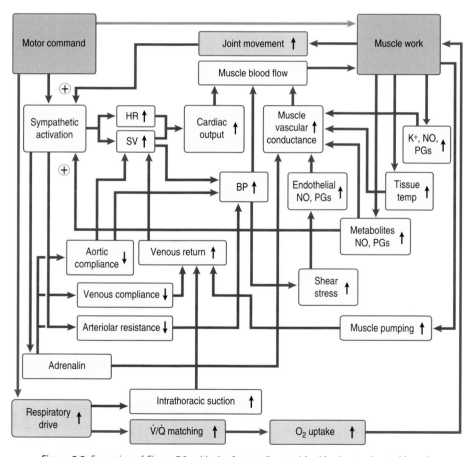

**Figure 8.3** Expansion of Figure 7.3, with the factors discussed in this chapter denoted in red.

matching, there is not enough time for equilibration of oxygen between alveolar air and bloodstream. In addition, they can be predicted to be relatively more susceptible to any circumstances that limit inspired oxygen levels, such as those associated with ascent to high altitude (see Chapter 12, p. 144). Some sports scientists have made the case that these athletes should be classified as having an abnormal arterial oxygenation response to exercise. A more realistic interpretation would be that they simply have an extremely efficient cardiovascular response.

## Case history

Robert A, a 42-year-old, non-obese man (76 kg) sought advice on an exercise training programme because he habitually became out of breath during quite moderate exertion. He thought that this might be due to lack of fitness. He had no history of major illness and appeared normal at rest, with no signs of breathlessness or cyanosis. At rest, resting heart rate was 74 beats/min and blood pressure 124/86 mmHg. Vital capacity was 4.8 l, tidal volume 750 ml, respiratory frequency 14 breaths/min. An attempt was made to measure his resting cardiac output by $CO_2$ Fick; end-expiratory $PCO_2$ was 26 mmHg and systemic venous $CO_2$ ($PvCO_2$) as measured by $CO_2$ rebreathing was 47 mmHg. Since this combination of values gave a calculated cardiac output far outside the normal range, a nitrous oxide rebreathing technique was used instead and gave a cardiac output of 5.6 l/min. Measurement of arterial oxygenation using a transcutaneous pulse oximeter on the earlobe showed saturation of 87% when breathing room air and 100% when breathing pure oxygen.

## Discussion

This case provides an opportunity for detailed reasoning about the coordination of respiratory function and the pulmonary circulation. First and most basically, Robert's arterial oxygen saturation was far lower than the 97–98% expected. This is likely to explain his low exercise tolerance, but what was the underlying reason? There was no obvious indication of abnormal cardiovascular or respiratory function. However, one dramatically abnormal set of data existed – while $PvCO_2$ was normal at 47 mmHg, end-expiratory $CO_2$, which should be identical to arterial $CO_2$ ($PaCO_2$) and, therefore, around 6 mmHg lower (41 mmHg), was in fact over 20 mmHg lower. This large blood–air difference could occur only if $CO_2$ was being expired more rapidly than normal by hyperventilation. Comparison of ventilatory and cardiovascular flows confirms this. Cardiac output was 5.6 l/min and, with a normal $\dot{V}/\dot{Q}$ ratio of 1.0, minute ventilation would be expected to be similar in magnitude. In fact, however, minute ventilation was (0.75.14) or 10.5 l/min.

This degree of hyperventilation might be expected as a result of peripheral chemoreceptor activation, since Robert's arterial oxygen saturation of 87% equates to a $PaO_2$ of around 60 mmHg – but what was the cause of the poor oxygenation? It could be because a proportion of the pulmonary vasculature was not perfused and the entire right cardiac output supplied a reduced volume of lung. This would increase the velocity of capillary blood flow and so reduce the time available for oxygen uptake. Alternatively, a proportion of the alveoli might not be ventilated, so that blood passing through some pulmonary capillaries remained unoxygenated. These possibilities can be distinguished by breathing pure oxygen. If the limitation is time for oxygen uptake, then this would be overcome by increasing the diffusional concentration gradient. On the other hand, dilution of normal arterial blood by deoxygenated blood returning from unventilated lung would persist regardless of efficiency of oxygen uptake in the remaining areas. In Robert's case, the data clearly indicated presence of an unperfused area of lung.

Subsequent radiological investigation showed that he had a long-standing thrombus lodged in his left pulmonary artery, so that his entire cardiac output was routed through the right half of his lung. With this knowledge it is easy to see why Robert's resting minute ventilation was around twice normal – he had to inspire twice as much as normal in order to provide adequate blood oxygenation. It is also clear why he became breathless during exercise. The need to move twice as much air as normal in and out of the lungs would cause respiratory muscle fatigue at lower levels of exercise. As well, routing all of the right cardiac output through only half of the pulmonary capillaries increases capillary transit speed and so lowers the safety margin for equilibration of oxygen between air and plasma when cardiac output rises with exercise. If $PaO_2$ falls far enough to activate hypoxia receptors, then there will be further respiratory muscle fatigue.

## PRACTICAL CONSEQUENCES OF LOW PULMONARY ARTERIAL PRESSURE

In addition to the functional considerations that we have examined in the previous sections of this chapter, the fact that pulmonary pressures and resistance are so much lower than those in the systemic circulation has two practical implications for the experimental physiologist.

### Kinetic pressure

In Chapter 3 (p. 28), we saw that intravascular pressures measured in the moving bloodstream can have a component that is due to the kinetic energy of fluid movement, depending on the orientation of the catheter tip. The value of this kinetic pressure is around 5 mmHg at rest, which is only a minor contribution to the total pressure in the systemic circulation. It is, on the other hand, a substantial proportion of pulmonary arterial pressure and very different values for pulmonary blood pressure would be recorded if a catheter had an end-opening or a side-opening tip. Remember also that the magnitude of the kinetic pressure component rises dramatically as cardiac output rises. If one is interpreting data on pulmonary pressures, especially during exercise, it is, therefore, important to know which catheter type was used, and it is equally important for the catheter type to be standardized between experiments where one wishes to compare pulmonary pressures.

## Pulmonary wedge pressure

If a pressure-sensing catheter with an open tip is introduced into the pulmonary artery through the right heart, it can be advanced down the arterial tree until it is wedged in one of the small arteries. Under these circumstances the catheter tip is sealed off from the arterial pressure upstream and the pressure recorded is that in the vessels downstream. But there is hardly any vascular resistance between the recording site and the final entry of pulmonary veins into the left atrium, so the pressure measured actually approximates left atrial pressure.

Recording of this so-called *wedge pressure* is the only practicable way in which mechanical function in the left heart can be measured, because it is not technically possible to pass a catheter retrogradely up the aorta and back into the heart. In practice, the catheter used for recording wedge pressure (called a *Swann-Ganz catheter*) has a small balloon just behind the tip that can be inflated so as to guarantee that the wedged tip is isolated from the pressure upstream (Fig. 8.4).

## IMPLICATIONS OF DEVELOPMENTAL CHANGES IN PULMONARY PERFUSION

Before birth, all foetal gas exchange takes place in the placenta where foetal venous and maternal arterial bloodstreams are separated only by thin membranes. As well, the foetal lungs are filled with relatively hypoxic amniotic fluid, so that the pulmonary microcirculation is compressed externally and

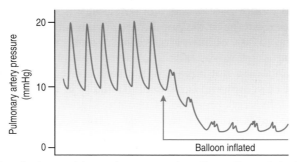

**Figure 8.4** Recording of pulmonary intravascular pressure using a Swann-Ganz catheter. Initially, pulmonary arterial pressure was recorded as 20/10 mmHg. At the arrow, the catheter balloon was inflated, sealing off the pressure-sensing catheter tip from the arterial inflow. Note the cessation of arterial pulsation and its replacement by typical atrial pulse waves with an absolute mean pressure around 4 mmHg.

is also constricted by activation of airways hypoxia receptors. At this time, therefore, the pulmonary circulation not only has no functional role, but also is a site of much higher vascular resistance than is the situation after birth. This creates higher systolic pressures in the fetal right atrium and ventricle, and pulmonary arteries than those in the corresponding parts of the left circulation. To prevent massive overwork of the right-side myocardium, most of the right cardiac output has to be short-circuited around the pulmonary circuit.

The shunting takes place in two ways (Moore 2003). The embryonic heart has only one atrium and one ventricle, which by around 8 weeks' gestation has been partitioned into left and right sides by formation of intervening walls. The inter-atrial wall grows from both upper and lower extremities of the common atrium, with the two leaves overlapping each other but not fusing. This forms a valve (called the *foramen ovale*) by which a proportion of the venous blood returning to the right atrium can flow directly into the left atrium. The second shunting pathway is a short, muscular blood vessel that runs between the aortic arch and the pulmonary artery and is known as the *ductus arteriosus*. This vessel is maintained in a dilated state during fetal life by cells in its wall synthesizing large amounts of relaxant prostaglandins. In consequence, all of the relatively small right stroke volume of blood that was not shunted through the foramen ovale flows from pulmonary artery to aorta, bypassing the pulmonary microcirculation.

At birth, both of these shunts cease to function as a result of the baby beginning to breathe. Expansion of the lungs with air removes both the compressive forces and the effect of hypoxia receptor stimulation. The consequent reduction in pulmonary vascular resistance reverses the pressure gradients between the atria, sealing the foramen ovale, and across the ductus arteriosus, which now carries oxygenated blood from aorta to pulmonary artery. Because the process of prostaglandin synthesis that held the ductus open before birth is efficient only in a hypoxic environment, perfusion by oxygenated blood causes ductus closure and terminates the shunt.

Over the next few days after birth, both shunts normally become sealed permanently by growth of new tissue. Nonetheless, this is not absolute in a surprisingly high percentage of the population. The foramen ovale does not seal completely in up to 30% of individuals and, in a much smaller percentage of people, the ductus arteriosus fails to close completely. The residual hole is usually small and may not have any noticeable effect on cardiorespiratory efficiency. Lack of symptoms is particularly likely in the case of the foramen ovale because left atrial pressure is usually higher than that in the right atrium so the shunt is normally held shut. However, if pulmonary vascular resistance rises then there is the potential for right–left shunting and reduced pulmonary perfusion.

With any persistent ductus arteriosus and with some cases of persistent foramen ovale, there is chronic left–right shunting resulting in right heart overload. Intense exercise may not be advisable in such individuals and will certainly not be associated with entirely normal cardiorespiratory responses to exercise. The presence of these abnormalities is very likely to cause systolic murmurs and so, even though they are rare, checking for murmurs is a sensible safeguard in any naïve subject being admitted to an exercise study. The Case History in Chapter 12 (p. 151) returns to this theme.

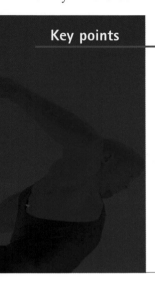

## Key points

The low pulmonary resistance is responsible for several important properties of the right-side circulation. While these save metabolic energy under normal circumstances they can result in inefficient cardiorespiratory function if pulmonary resistance is increased.

At rest, the matching of ventilation and perfusion varies dramatically in different regions of the lung.

With increasing intensity of aerobic exercise this variation progressively disappears.

Shunting between right- and left-side circulations is an essential feature of the foetal circulation and persistence of these after birth is relatively common, and may interfere with exercise capacity.

## References

Moore KL, Persaud TVN 2003 Before we are born, 6th edn, Saunders, Philadelphia, Chapter 15.
Moudgil R, Michelakis ED, Archer SL 2005 Hypoxic pulmonary vasoconstriction. Journal of Applied Physiology 98: 390–403.

## Further reading

Stewart IB, Pickering RL 2006 Effect of prolonged exercise on arterial oxygen saturation in athletes susceptible to exercise-induced hypoxemia. Scandinavian Journal of Medicine and Science in Sports 17: 445–451.

### Questions for revision

- Discuss the functional consequences of the fact that pulmonary vascular resistance is around one-seventh that of the systemic circulation.

- Why does the ventilation/perfusion ratio vary between different regions of the lung at rest?

- What processes cause the ventilation/perfusion ratio to become more evenly distributed across all regions of the lung during exercise?

- Discuss the reasons that right–left shunting is essential in the foetal circulation and indicate the locations of these shunts.

# Chapter 9

# Circulatory limits to acute exercise

## CHAPTER CONTENTS

### After reading this chapter, you should:

- appreciate that exercise performance is normally limited by cardiovascular factors
- know how to assess fluid loss by sweating and how to optimize exercise capacity by limiting fluid depletion
- understand the impact of body size, gender and age on exercise performance
- recognize the particular limitations to cardiovascular servicing of exercise capacity that are imposed by different environments

Dynamic work capacity is proportional to the amount of aerobic metabolism that can take place in the cells of the locomotor skeletal muscles. Although the efficiency of these metabolic processes can be manipulated by, for example, dietary selection so as to optimize the appropriate substrates and training-induced adaptation of muscle fibre type, the end result is a reflection of oxygen availability. As such, the primary limit to exercise is the rate at which oxygen can be delivered to the muscle.

As discussed in Chapter 8 (p. 99), ventilatory function and pulmonary oxygen uptake in the pulmonary capillaries are not normally limiting factors since, even at peak workloads, arterial oxygen saturation is similar to that at rest, except in the subset of elite athletes with exceptional cardiac adaptations to training. However, we saw in Chapter 3 that the volume of blood that can be pumped around the circulation per unit time is determined by the age-limited maximum heart rate and by the decline in ventricular filling at high heart rates. These changes set an absolute limit of around 0.3 l/min/kg to cardiac output in an untrained individual, equating to around 21 l/min in a 70 kg person. The purpose of the current chapter is to examine in detail the factors that limit cardiac output at different exercise durations and intensities, under different environmental circumstances and in relation to different types of individual.

## FACTORS THAT LIMIT MUSCLE PERFUSION

### Effects of exercise hyperaemia

In resting muscle, where there is a relatively high precapillary vasoconstrictor tone, mean capillary hydrostatic pressure and plasma oncotic pressure are both around 25 mmHg, so that there is a balance between inwardly and outwardly directed pressure gradients and no net water movement occurs across the capillary wall. When the muscle arterioles dilate with onset of exercise, however, the resulting fall in precapillary resistance automatically raises capillary hydrostatic pressure, to values as high as 50–60 mmHg when the arterioles are maximally dilated. Because this is far above the opposing oncotic pressure value, net extravasation of plasma water takes place until the resultant increase in interstitial hydrostatic pressure is sufficient to rebalance the outward/inward forces (Fortney et al 1981). At least at high muscle workloads, the outward water movement is increased further by the rise in interstitial osmolality caused by accumulation of muscle metabolites.

Since skeletal muscle makes up such a large proportion of total body mass, the volume of extravasated fluid within the muscles during whole-body dynamic exercise can be appreciable. At relatively heavy workloads, 10–12% of plasma volume (around 300 ml in a 70 kg person) is lost over the initial 10 min of activity (Fig. 9.1). Thus, over this period cardiac output also falls by around 300 ml provided heart rate remains constant, necessarily reducing muscle blood flow. Moreover, plasma loss results in a concomitant rise in haematocrit, elevating blood viscosity and so increasing cardiac workload.

### Effect of heat production

Muscle activity generates metabolic heat and, therefore, potentially elevates core body temperature. Even at high work intensities, it takes at least several minutes for this heat to diffuse into the circulation and be detected by the hypothalamic thermostat. The initial stage of exercise is, therefore, independent of thermoregulatory considerations. As soon as cardiac output is warmed by more than around 0.01° C, however, compensatory heat loss processes begin to be activated. These impose new, increasingly severe limitations on the amount of blood available for muscle perfusion.

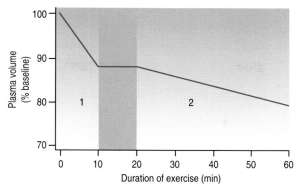

**Figure 9.1** Typical timecourse of plasma volume reduction during maintained exercise. Note the rapid fall due to muscle extravasation (1) and the slower decline associated with sweating (2). The delayed onset of pronounced sweating reflects the time taken for metabolic heat to accumulate in muscle and to diffuse from muscle to bloodstream.

As mentioned in Chapter 6 (p. 68), the first of these processes is withdrawal of sympathetic vasoconstrictor tone from the cutaneous arterioles. In parallel, there is activation of cholinergic sympathetic nerves to eccrine sweat glands. Both the loss of sympathetic tone and the process of sweat production cause cutaneous vasodilation. As a result, skin blood flow rises from a resting value that is typically less than 500 ml/min at environmental temperatures below 25° C to as much as 3 l/min after 15–20 min of sustained heavy exercise, with a similar fall in muscle blood flow. The dilatation due to sweating is at least partly secondary to glandular release of kinins (see Chapter 6, p. 75) but may also involve release of unknown dilator factors from the sudomotor nerve endings (Joyner & Halliwill 2000). As well as serving to convey heat to the body/environment interface, the high skin blood flow is essential to provide water and electrolytes for sweat production. This typically reaches a maximum of around 1 l/h, but may be as high as 2 l/h in a person who exercises routinely in hot conditions.

Sweating produces a second phase of plasma volume reduction that typically becomes measurable around 20 min after commencement of exercise (Fig. 9.1). Although in theory plasma and interstitial fluids are in equilibrium, high rates of sweat production draw primarily on the plasma, so that blood volume falls and haematocrit rises progressively as the exercise bout continues. Both effects make muscle oxygenation progressively more and more inefficient.

## Measurement of sweating

A wide range of techniques are available for measuring sweat production, but none are suitable for all applications. Choice of technique depends critically on the intensity of sweat secretion to be measured and the duration of measurement required. All techniques in routine use involve one of four basic principles, as summarized below.

### Skin resistance

The superficial layer of the skin consists of non-nucleated cells whose cytoplasm has been replaced by keratin. The absence of cellular water and electrolytes makes this layer of skin a good insulator with extremely high resistance to passage of electrical current. As the sweat ducts fill during sweat secretion, a low-resistance pathway is established between the internal and external surfaces of the skin. Skin resistance can easily be measured by passing a low DC current (3–4V) between an ECG electrode that is in electrical continuity with the body interior and an electrode placed on the skin surface. It is possible to obtain instantaneous indices of sweat production at various sites by applying the surface electrode manually or to have a continuous record of sweating at one site by using a stationary surface electrode.

The most dramatic change in skin resistance occurs between the states of non-sweating and of slow sweating, reflecting the process of initially overcoming the almost complete insulation of the skin. This technique is, therefore, extremely good for ascertaining the time of onset of sweating; for example, during a timed period of exercise at a specific intensity. Once the skin surface is wet with sweat, on the other hand, it is not possible to obtain quantitative information on the volume of sweat produced.

### Detection of moisture

Certain chemical compounds have the property of changing colour when they absorb water and this can be used to detect whether the skin is dry or wet. The compound of usual choice is cobalt chloride, which is blue when dry and pink when hydrated. In practice, strips of stiff absorbent paper (such as Whatman no. 1 filter paper) are dipped in a 1% solution of cobalt chloride, dried and stored in a dessicator. In order to determine the time of onset of sweating, strips are pressed briefly against an identifiable area of skin at regular intervals, and arrival of sweat at the mouths of individual sweat ducts will be seen as punctate pink spots.

At low sweat rates, this technique is also able to quantify sweat secretion by measuring the size of the spots manually or, more easily, in a densitometric image analyzer. At relatively high rates of sweating, by contrast, the entire skin surface is moist and so no gradation of colour exists.

### Volume collection

Except in very humid environments, sweat evaporates rapidly from the skin, even at quite high rates of secretion. If, however, a container is placed on the skin surface so as to prevent evaporative loss, then the sweat produced over that area of skin will be retained and can be measured. For obvious reasons, this technique cannot be used to detect the onset of sweating and is not practicable with very low sweat rates. But at high rates of production it can provide accurate quantitative values, provided that evaporative loss is prevented during the process of measurement and that the duration of collection is appropriate for the volume of the sampling vessel. One advantage of this method is the capacity to make repeated measurements for the same set of sweat glands over a prolonged period. A limitation is the lack of information obtained on behaviour of sweat glands elsewhere on the body.

## Body mass

At relatively high rates of whole-body sweat secretion, the amount of sweat produced can be determined by the loss of body mass. Obvious precautions needed are monitoring of any fluid intake or urinary output and measurement of nude body mass in order to include loss of the sweat trapped in clothing. Given that most electronic balances capable of measuring body mass cannot detect changes less than 50 g, this technique is not practicable at low rates of sweating. During intense exercise or other types of severe thermal stress, by contrast, when sweat production is typically at least 1 l (1 kg)/h, it is possible to make repeated measurements with a high degree of accuracy at intervals of 10–15 min.

### HANDY HINTS

Since maintaining cardiac output during sustained exercise depends on effective replacement of the fluid volume that is lost through sweating, it is worth considering how to optimize this replacement. Taking the case of moderate exercise in a warm environment, the volume of sweat lost might be of the order of 0.5 l/h and, in a subject who is not heat-acclimatized, each litre of sweat will contain about 2.5 g (half a teaspoon) sodium chloride.

Two factors have to be considered when replacing this fluid. Gastric emptying will be facilitated by drinking relatively small volumes (not more than 100–200 ml) frequently and by ensuring the fluid is cool but not ice-cold. Intestinal absorption will be facilitated by ensuring that the osmotic gradient encourages water movement into the blood stream; in other words that the ingested fluid is hypotonic. A solution that matches the sweat lost by containing 2.5 g salt/l represents 0.25% saline. This has a much lower osmolality than the 0.9% saline that is isotonic with plasma.

Addition of a small amount of glucose, around 20 g (2 tablespoons)/l, will speed up absorption further. This activates the intestinal glucose/sodium co-transporter, while still providing a total osmolality that is well below that of plasma.

## Heart rate drift

During sustained dynamic exercise, heart rate begins to drift upwards from its previously stable level. The drift is prevented almost entirely by adequate fluid replacement during exercise, confirming that it involves reflex sympathetic compensation for the progressive fall in circulating plasma volume. In addition, prolonged muscle activity tends to involve progressive recruitment of larger numbers of muscle units as compensation for fatigue of those first recruited. Since greater descending motor drive is associated with greater activation of the cardiovascular centre, this also increases cardiac sympathetic drive.

The functional consequence of heart rate drift is further encroachment on ventricular filling time, introducing another factor that acts to limit muscle perfusion. Heart rate drift also needs to be borne in mind when absolute heart rate is being used to set training intensity, since 30 min whole-body activity at intensities of 80% or higher is associated typically with a drift of up to 15 beats/min.

## Competition with other metabolically active tissues

Consideration of partitioning of cardiac output during exercise usually assumes that the only significant competition occurs between locomotor muscle and skin circulations, as discussed above. There are, however, two situations in which additional competitions must be considered.

One of these is that, in large-bodied, highly trained athletes, the metabolic demand of the respiratory muscles can be a potential limiting factor in locomotor muscle perfusion during intense activity (Dempsey et al 2006). In other subjects the amount of tissue involved is not sufficient to impose a significant perfusional load but, even so, it is possible that chemoreceptor inputs from metabolite build-up in respiratory muscles may contribute to the sensation of fatigue during intense activity.

Second, although the exercise response relies on increased, sympathetically mediated peripheral resistance in the splanchnic circulation, this is effective only while the metabolic rate of the splanchnic tissues remains low. Ingestion of a substantial meal within 1–2 h of exercise will activate gastric, hepatic and intestinal metabolism, and the associated splanchnic hyperaemia due to release of local metabolites and hormones must limit the absolute blood flow available to active skeletal muscles. More importantly, because skeletal muscle and splanchnic beds are the two regions that contribute most to peripheral resistance changes during regulation of blood pressure, overriding sympathetic tone in both of them simultaneously makes it extremely difficult to maintain a blood pressure gradient adequate for effective muscle perfusion.

Figure 9.2 adds these limiting factors to our flow chart of the matrix of responses to exercise.

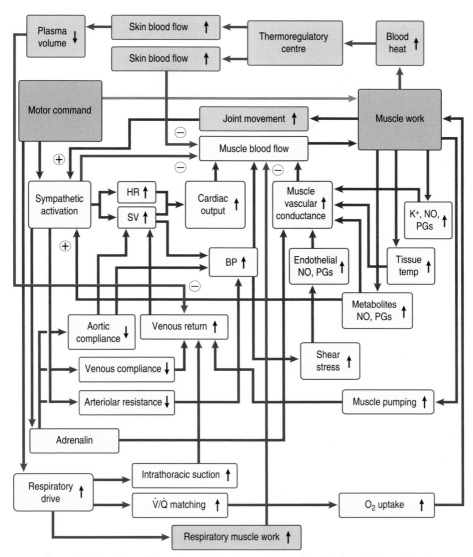

**Figure 9.2** Expansion of Figure 8.3, with the factors discussed in this chapter denoted in red.

# EFFECTS OF DIFFERENT ENVIRONMENTS

## Temperature and humidity

Since the need for heat loss imposes major limitations on muscle blood flow, it is predictable that environments that affect thermoregulatory efficiency will influence exercise capacity. Thus, time to fatigue is increased under cold conditions due to both reduced skin blood flow and sweating (Blanchet et al 2003). During rapid exposure to a very cold environment (such as on immersion in cold water) there is profound cutaneous vasoconstriction that can result in dramatic elevation of blood pressure and it is possible that, even with less extreme activation of skin cold receptors, the pressure gradient for muscle perfusion during exercise will be somewhat higher than under thermoneutral conditions. It is, however, not known whether this has any real effect on the efficiency of muscle perfusion.

The redistribution of cardiac output associated with reduced cutaneous perfusion leads to increased renal blood flow, glomerular filtration and urine formation (*cold diuresis*). In addition, the reduced humidity of cold air means that there is an increase in evaporative water loss associated with ventilation. While these factors provide additional sources of fluid loss during prolonged exercise, effective blood volume is usually conserved by the lower rate of sweating.

In cold environments, other issues that combine circulatory and thermoregulatory considerations may complicate the situation further. Thus, varying efficiencies of insulative clothing may create microenvironments that range from one that tends towards producing hypothermia due to evaporative and convective cooling to one that retards heat loss so much that it produces hyperthermia. In addition, extreme cold especially in windy conditions can overwhelm the cold dilator response that normally protects digits, ears and nose (see Chapter 5, p. 58) and result in freezing of cells in these tissues (*frostbite*).

Hot environments will reduce time to fatigue because of greater skin blood flow and of more rapid depletion of plasma volume by sweating. In addition, environmental humidity has a profound influence because it dictates the efficiency of sweat evaporation. Under conditions of high relative humidity, evaporation may be virtually eliminated and so sweating produces no heat loss. In response, sweat production is increased. This may result in maximal sweat production and substantial plasma volume loss (up to 2 l/h) at work rates that would, under dry conditions, produce only trivial sweating.

Even without taking into consideration the progressive encroachment on circulatory performance caused by hot conditions, absolute exercise capacity is lower in the heat. Expansion of vascular volume caused by generalized dilation of the cutaneous veins reduces venous return and so lowers stroke volume. As a result, maximal heart rate is reached at a cardiac output that may be as little as 80% of that achieved under thermoneutral conditions, and maximum work capacity is reduced correspondingly.

## Aquatic vs. terrestrial exercise

The relative inefficiency of swimming due to the high density of the medium is to some extent countered by the absence of some of the problems that limit terrestrial exercise. The high thermal conductivity of water means that heat loss occurs very rapidly and without the need for massive cutaneous vasodilation or sweating. As well, effective circulating blood volume is increased, both by lack of gravitational pooling and by the fact that the external pressure of the water compresses the superficial veins. Together, these factors allow muscle perfusion to be a higher proportion of cardiac output than during terrestrial activity and for it to be maintained stable for far longer periods.

Breath-hold swimming underwater triggers a unique pattern of reflex cardiovascular changes, consisting of bradycardia and a generalized increase in peripheral resistance that includes vasoconstriction of skeletal muscle blood vessels. Extensive experimentation has shown that in diving animals, such as seals, this so-called *diving response* can produce heart rates as low as 5–10 beats/min, with almost complete cessation of blood flow through the exercising skeletal muscles. This reduces dramatically the rate of oxygen consumption and carbon dioxide production and allows these animals to undertake dives that may last for more than 30 min. In man, the diving response is much less pronounced.

Specialized diving species have powerful sympathetic innervation of the larger arteries supplying limb muscles, so they can shut off blood flow external to the muscles. By contrast, blood flow to exercising muscles in man falls only moderately because the vasoconstrictor innervation is localized to the microcirculation within the muscle, so its effect is opposed by the vasodilator effect of local metabolites. As a result, muscle perfusion and consequent build-up of carbon dioxide in the bloodstream cannot be avoided, and breath-holding is possible for only 1–2 min at most before arterial hypercapnia activates the central chemoreceptors and produces an irresistible urge to breathe.

## EFFECTS OF GENDER

Regardless of fitness level, maximal work capacity in women is always around 20% less than in men of the same age. This is due in part to the fact that testosterone and oestrogens exert differential effects on the growth of muscle and fat cells, so that muscle always constitutes a smaller proportion of body mass in women. However, cardiovascular factors also play a major part in the gender difference. Testosterone stimulates erythropoiesis, so that men have haematocrits that are on average 10% higher than those in women and, therefore, have greater capacities to carry oxygen in any given cardiac output. In addition, men have larger hearts relative to body mass, so they can produce greater stroke volumes and, therefore, greater maximum perfusion per unit mass of muscle.

## EFFECTS OF AGE

### Children

#### Cardiovascular factors

The cardiovascular systems of children and adolescents differ quantitatively from those of adults in several ways that impact on the response to exercise.

First, children have lower heart sizes than adults relative to body mass, so their stroke volumes are lower. At any age, heart mass and stroke volume are slightly lower in girls than in boys. While heart size rises with age, stroke volume remains less than that in adults until late adolescence. In addition, studies that have investigated responses to maximum exercise in children and adolescents have been unable to show that the ceiling heart rate is significantly higher than the 200 beats/min typical of a 20-year-old (see Chapter 3, p. 20). Therefore, the relatively low stroke volumes in children mean that given increments of cardiac output require greater increments in heart rate than in adults, and the maximal cardiac output that can be achieved must be assumed to be lower than that in adults.

Nonetheless, there is more variability in maximum heart rate among children of any age than would be seen in adults and some children show maxima as high as 220 beats/min (Dencker et al 2006). On the basis of these findings it has been suggested that the true maximum rate is, in fact, greater than in adults and that failure to see this consistently is because children are often not motivated to reach their true maximum workload during testing. At present, the situation remains unresolved but, in the absence of an alternate consensus view, it is safest to assume that age-related changes in maximum heart rate begin only after adolescence.

A further difference between children and adults is that children of both sexes below the age of puberty have haematocrits that are slightly lower than those after puberty, at around 36–38%. Intuitively, the combination of lower cardiac output and lower oxygen carrying capacity would be thought to limit exercise in children. Nonetheless, these differences appear to confer little or no cardiovascular disadvantage on the capacity of children to produce short-term aerobic work, because they have greater capacity than adults for oxygen extraction in exercising muscles (Turley & Wilmore 1997). The mechanisms underlying this are not certain. Probable contributing factors include differences in muscle cell metabolism and the fact that smaller muscles have shorter diffusional distances between plasma and muscle cell.

## Thermoregulatory factors

Thermoregulatory limitations also impinge on exercise capacity in children. In the cold, children are less well equipped than adults to maintain homeothermy. This is because of the greater heat loss associated with a greater surface area:body mass ratio and with reduced insulative adiposity. In the heat, their lower capacity to increase cardiac output means that partitioning of blood flows between muscle and skin becomes a limiting factor in muscle perfusion with smaller decrements in plasma volume. In addition, children have a lower capacity to produce eccrine sweat than adults and their sweating threshold is higher, so that sweat is at least in theory a less effective way of losing body heat.

Nonetheless, children appear to be at least as efficient as adults in maintaining body temperature during exercise in hot conditions (Inbar et al 2004). Their higher surface area:body mass ratio contributes to this. As well, the higher sweat rates seen in adults may not provide more effective evaporation because some of the sweat drips off the skin.

## Old age

Although the increasingly sedentary lifestyle that often accompanies ageing itself limits exercise, increasing age can also be shown to be associated with significant changes in cardiovascular correlates of exercise.

### Cardiovascular factors

Ageing is associated with progressive degradation of elastin elements in the connective tissues of all organ systems. In relation to cardiac function, this stiffens the ventricular walls and so reduces the efficiency of diastolic filling. As a result, stroke volume declines progressively with age, being by the age of 60 years only around 60% of the value in young adulthood. Despite this fall in stroke volume, resting heart rate remains unchanged, because the loss of muscle bulk and the increased mass of poorly perfused adipose tissue increase total peripheral resistance. Consequently, resting cardiac output falls in proportion to stroke volume, to around 3 l/min by age 60 in a 70 kg person.

The reduced stroke volume, together with the age-related fall in maximal heart rate, means that maximal cardiac output during exercise declines substantially with age. For example, an individual whose maximum output in young adulthood was (100 ml.200 beats/min) or 20 l/min can be expected at age 60 to generate a maximum output around ({60% of 100 ml}.[220–60] beats/min) or a little under 10 l/min.

Not only is maximum heart rate reduced with age but, in addition, the increment of tachycardia for any given submaximal workload is reduced, so that cardiac output falls relative to fractional work capacity. This change probably has several underlying mechanisms. Declining cardiac β-adrenoceptor sensitivity damps the sinoatrial response to sympathetic activation. Reduced muscle bulk may reduce the sensory inputs from muscle receptors that contribute to sympathetic drive. In addition, the loss of elastin from arterial vessels results in greater elevation of blood pressure during exercise. This may cause some baroreceptor-mediated inhibition of cardiac drive.

### Thermoregulatory factors

The elderly subject also faces additional thermoregulatory challenges during exercise. The lower absolute cardiac output imposes a stricter quota on partitioning of blood flows between muscle and skin as exercise progresses. Skin temperature rises more slowly during prolonged exercise, potentially limiting thermoregulatory stability. One reason for this is the overall increase in vascular resistance due to loss of elastic tissue, limiting skin blood flow. There is also evidence that ageing desensitizes the hypothalamic thermostatic centre, so that greater increments in blood temperature are required before heat loss processes are activated. Also, the gain of many autonomic reflexes falls with age, so that there may be less sudomotor discharge. Finally, atrophic changes in ageing skin are associated with decreased size of individual sweat glands.

## EFFECTS OF PREGNANCY

As pregnancy progresses, blood flow to the uterus and its contents rises to reach around 1 l/min at term. This does not detract from the amount of blood available to service exercise demands since over the same time-course blood volume rises by around 1.5 l. However, pregnancy does impose conditions that need to be considered as potential limiting factors in exercise capacity.

First, the additional mass imposed by the pregnant uterus will increase the absolute cardiac output and energy expenditure needed to produce a given amount of external work. Comparison of heart rate and oxygen consumption between pre-term and post-delivery has confirmed that the removal of the approximately 10 kg mass of foetus and placenta is associated with substantially less cardiovascular load in order to support a given intensity of submaximal exercise.

Second, the generalized sympathetic vasoconstriction of visceral beds that accompanies exercise may shunt blood away from the uterus and so reduce foetal oxygenation. In fact, although the uterine vasculature receives a powerful sympathetic innervation, this produces no effect on foetoplacental blood flow during pregnancy because the high local oestrogen and progesterone levels prevent vascular smooth muscle activation. Nonetheless, this safety mechanism is effective only when blood pressure remains adequate for optimal regional perfusion. When a woman in the last few months of pregnancy lies supine, the mass of the uterus is sufficient to compress the inferior vena cava, with significant falls in venous return, cardiac output and blood pressure. Weight-lifting on a bench or supine cycle ergometry may, therefore, reduce foetoplacental blood flow despite the local safety mechanisms.

Third, the additional heat load produced by the foetoplacental unit may result in body temperature rising more rapidly and further than normal during exercise. However, although the undoubted increase in absolute heat production during a given exercise intensity highlights potential dangers for intense exercise in hot environments, there is no good evidence of pregnant women being more susceptible to hyperthermia during moderate exercise in non-extreme environments. This is due probably to the vasodilator effect of oestrogens on skin blood vessels, together with the fact that progesterone raises the set point of the hypothalamic thermostat by around $0.5°$ C $(0.3°$ F), increasing the gradient for heat diffusion into the environment except at very high ambient temperatures.

Thus, there do not seem to be any contraindications to a pregnant woman performing exercise and the benefits of exercise in terms of musculoskeletal function make it generally advisable to undertake regular exercise until close to term. Apart from the cautions that need to be applied in relation to overheating, exercise such as running with an increased body mass has the potential to produce joint damage. Swimming is therefore often seen as the optimal pregnancy exercise modality, since it obviates both thermoregulatory and kinetic problems.

## Key points

The vasodilator effect of exercise in active skeletal muscle necessarily causes rapid depletion of effective plasma volume by 10–15%.

During prolonged activity, exercise capacity becomes increasingly limited by competition between muscle perfusion and thermoregulatory demands. The efficiency of exercise is, therefore, affected by environmental conditions.

Several techniques are available by which fluid loss by sweat production can be assessed. The choice of technique depends critically on the rate at which sweating is occurring.

Anatomical and physiological factors mean that absolute exercise capacity is less in women than in men and in children than in adults.

Exercise capacity declines with age, primarily reflecting the decline in maximum heart rate.

Because of the different cardiovascular adjustments that accompany terrestrial and aquatic exercise, swimming is the optimal exercise modality during pregnancy.

## References

Blanchet M, Ducharme A, Racine N et al 2003 Effects of cold exposure on submaximal exercise performance and adrenergic activation in patients with congestive heart failure and the effects of beta-adrenergic blockade (carvedilol or metoprolol). American Journal of Cardiology 92: 548–553.

Dempsey JA, Romer L, Rodman J, Miller J, Smith C 2006 Consequences of exercise-induced respiratory muscle work. Respiratory Physiology and Neurobiology 151: 242–250.

Dencker M, Thorsson O, Karlsson M et al 2006 Daily physical activity and its relation to physical fitness in children aged 8–11 years. European Journal of Applied Physiology 96: 587–592.

Fortney SM, Nadel ER, Wenger CB, Bove JR 1981 Effect of blood volume on sweating rate and body fluids in exercising humans. Journal of Applied Physiology 51: 1594–1600.

Inbar O, Morris N, Epstein Y, Gass G 2004 Comparison of thermoregulatory responses to exercise in dry heat among prepubertal boys, young adults and older males. Experimental Physiology 89: 691–700.

Joyner MJ, Halliwill JR 2000 Sympathetic vasodilatation in human limbs. Journal of Physiology 526: 471–480.

Turley KR, Wilmore JH 1997 Cardiovascular responses to treadmill and cycle ergometer exercise in children and adults. Journal of Applied Physiology 83: 948–957.

## Questions for revision

- Why does muscle blood flow decline during prolonged exercise at a given intensity?

- What techniques would be suitable for determining the time of onset of eccrine sweating during a 40 min period of sustained aerobic exercise?

- What is meant by 'heart rate drift' during prolonged exercise and to what is it due?

- Compare and contrast the cardiovascular limitations to exercise capacity in children, young adults and the elderly.

- What considerations need to be taken into account when recommending regular exercise during pregnancy?

# Chapter 10

# Adverse circulatory effects of exercise

## CHAPTER CONTENTS

### After reading this chapter, you should:

- appreciate the different ways in which fainting (syncope) may be produced during exercise
- understand the potentially adverse effects of exercise on body temperature and body fluid content and composition
- know the principles of how to deal with these problems
- be able to identify some specific situations in which exercise may be life-threatening

## SYNCOPE

In an upright individual, the gravitational field between heart and brain means that cerebral perfusion pressure is always lower than blood pressure at the level of the arterial baroreceptors. In consequence, cerebral perfusion varies more dramatically with variations in cardiac ejection and peripheral resistance than does perfusion to other organs, and situations that result in substantially reduced blood pressure may, in the upright posture, result in fainting (*syncope*) due to inadequate blood flow to the forebrain.

### Causes of syncope

Such reductions in blood pressure could result from reduced venous return and cardiac filling or from reduced baroreflex capacity to induce peripheral

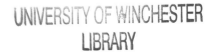

vasoconstriction. In the context of exercise, the typical primary effect is obstructed systemic venous return due to elevation of intrathoracic pressure. This pressure increase can be induced voluntarily by forced expiration against a closed glottis and is known as the *Valsalva manoeuvre* (Fig. 10.1). It occurs naturally during any activity that involves thoracic muscle activation and breath holding, such as carrying heavy suitcases, weight lifting or straining on the lavatory.

In normal, healthy individuals, the arterial baroreflex responses to reduced stroke volume (increased peripheral resistance and tachycardia) are usually fast and large enough to maintain blood pressure at a level that allows adequate cerebral perfusion. Several factors can, however, reduce the effectiveness of these compensations so that consciousness is impaired. Reduced blood volume will reduce the efficiency of cardiac filling and so exaggerate the fall in stroke volume. Increased venous compliance will lead to greater pooling of blood in dependent veins, with less efficient mobilization of this for any given degree of sympathetic vasoconstrictor activation. Finally, any blood-borne influences that cause cerebral vasoconstriction will reduce cerebral perfusion further at any given blood pressure.

All of these additional factors may be associated with athletic performance of specific types. In competitions that involve weight divisions, many performers restrict their fluid intake dramatically in order to make weight, with resulting depletion of plasma volume. Intense, long-term dynamic training has been reported to cause increases in compliance of the large veins, predisposing these athletes to increased venous pooling and to hypotension and fainting during rapid postural change, even in the absence of a Valsalva

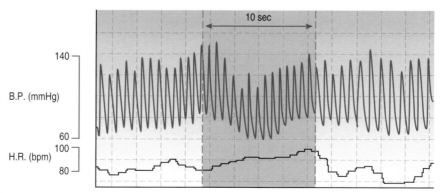

**Figure 10.1** Effects on blood pressure and heart rate of 10 s forced expiration against a resistance of 44 mHg, in a young, healthy adult. During the Valsalva manoeuvre, reduced venous return is compensated by increased sympathetic vasoconstriction and tachycardia, which together restore mean blood pressure near to the pre-test value. The fact that this restoration is not complete until near the end of the manoeuvre reflects the slow time course of vascular smooth muscle contraction following sympathetic activation. This is mirrored by the relative bradycardia that occurs over the 10 s after cessation of the manoeuvre and reflects the bradycardic baroreflex response to elevated peripheral resistance.

manoeuvre (Hernandez & Franke 2004). Finally, the elevation of plasma adrenaline (epinephrine) and noradrenaline (norepinephrine) due to the generalized sympathetic discharge associated with central command is enhanced by the additional sympathetic activation due to the stress of competition. Although the cerebral vasculature itself receives only a sparse sympathetic innervation, these circulating catecholamines exert a moderate vasoconstrictor effect on the cerebral precapillary resistance vessels and so reduce brain perfusion at any given level of pressure gradient. An example of Valsalva-induced syncope in a competitive athlete appears in the Case history below.

## Case history

Joe K, a competitive weight lifter, was preparing for the national championships, but was having difficulty in making the weight for the 69 kg (152.1 lb) division. Three days before weigh-in he was still several kg heavier than necessary and he just managed to achieve 69 kg by severely limiting his fluid intake. In competition, he was confident enough to pass on the initial round and then made his first snatch satisfactorily. But during the final phase of his first clean and jerk he suddenly became dizzy, collapsed and had to withdraw.

## Comment

Weight lifting, along with many other forms of static and resistive exercises involving the upper body, necessarily causes a very substantial increase in intrathoracic pressure. This is equivalent to a Valsalva manoeuvre and consequently reduces venous return, stroke volume and blood pressure.

In Joe's case, several interactive factors were probably involved in the Valsalva manoeuvre during competition producing such a severe fall in blood pressure that he lost consciousness. First, his restricted fluid intake prior to competition would have lowered his plasma volume and reduced the amount of blood that could be mobilized from his dependent veins during sympathetic venoconstriction. Second, the stress of competition leads to elevated circulating catecholamines, which will exert some constrictor effect on the cerebral arterioles. Third, most weight lifters hyperventilate immediately before a lift. This produces hypocapnia, which lowers the cerebral interstitial proton concentration. Protons constitute the single most powerful metabolic dilator influence on the cerebral arterioles, so hypocapnia causes significant cerebral vasoconstriction.

## HYPERTHERMIA

### Dependence on evaporative cooling

As discussed in Chapter 9 (p. 106), the internal heat generated by even intense prolonged exercise produces only moderate hyperthermia, so long as there is effective evaporative cooling by sweat. By definition, therefore, anything that interferes with heat loss is likely to result in excessive elevation of body temperature. If this rises to more than 41° C (106° F) then central nervous function begins to be impaired, with permanent brain damage or death occurring at only slightly higher temperatures.

Sweat is a highly effective source of heat loss when air humidity is low. This is illustrated dramatically by our capacity to maintain a near-normal core temperature in sauna baths, where the temperature is routinely set at around 100° C (212° F), but relative humidity is around 10% or less. However, the efficiency of evaporative heat loss is highly dependent on absolute relative humidity, as witnessed by the greatly increased sweat production produced by quite small increments in sauna humidity when one pours water on the coals. If environmental relative humidity is 90% or more, as is often the case in many tropical climates, then virtually no sweat evaporates and there is consequently almost no benefit for heat loss, despite the fact that the volume of sweat secreted for a given workload and ambient temperature is much greater than under less humid conditions (Fig. 10.2). Under these circumstances, heat loss depends almost entirely on radiation and convection, which are far less efficient than evaporation.

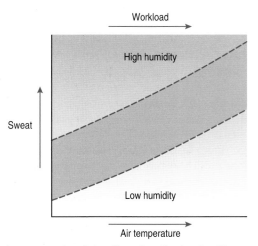

**Figure 10.2** Diagrammatic representation of the effect of workload and ambient temperature on sweat production under conditions of low or high relative humidity. Note that for any given workload and air temperature, sweat production is higher in humid than in dry conditions.

# Heat exhaustion

In the absence of fluid replacement, plasma volume falls during exercise in line with the volume of sweat produced. Below a critical volume, it becomes impossible to maintain blood pressure in the face of the overall low peripheral resistance imposed by dilatation in muscle and cutaneous beds. As a result, cerebral perfusion is prejudiced in the upright posture and the individual collapses. The time to onset of this state of *heat exhaustion* will be determined primarily by the rate of sweating and, therefore, depends on workload and on environmental temperature and humidity. Under competitive conditions, it can also be prolonged by motivation, to the extent that collapse does not occur until fluid depletion is so great that sweat production has begun to decline.

Since evaporative heat loss continues to be effective until at least shortly before onset of heat exhaustion, core temperature at the time of collapse from heat exhaustion is normal or only slightly elevated. However, it may rise more dramatically after collapse. Cessation of limb movement reduces convective and radiative heat loss, and even after muscle activity stops there is a large residual store of metabolic heat in the previously active muscle mass. Particularly when sweating is already decreased by fluid depletion, these factors can elevate core temperature to dangerously high levels.

# Heat stroke

With normal evaporative heat loss, as discussed above, core temperature can be held close to the resting value even during intense work in hot environments, provided that plasma volume is maintained. If the efficiency of the evaporative heat loss pathway is impaired, however, exercise in the heat may elevate core temperature rapidly to values in excess of 40° C (104° F), resulting in *heat stroke*. Initially there is confusion, with reduced capacity for cognition and decision-making and at internal temperatures of around 41.5° C (107° F) consciousness is lost. At 42° C (108° F), sustained and often fatal damage to central neuronal structures occurs due to protein coagulation.

Individuals most susceptible to heat stroke during physical activity are, predictably, those in whom heat loss is minimized by insulative clothing and who are compelled to maintain a high level of work in a hot environment. Typical examples of this group are soldiers on route march and grid-iron footballers. As well, as discussed in the preceding section, it is important to remember that even when exercise stops heat will continue to enter the bloodstream from the previously active muscles. In situations of severe hyperthermia, where very small increments of core temperature can mean the difference between life and death, immediate and efficient removal of heat from the body is essential.

Because there is only a narrow range between normothermia and the temperature at which irreversible cerebral protein damage occurs, it is essential to halt the rise in core temperature rapidly. The obvious first step is to shelter the victim from solar heat gain. The next is to provide effective pathways for heat loss.

With core temperatures that are not higher than 40° C (104° F), copious sponging of the skin with water is usually effective, provided that the environment is relatively dry. At temperatures closer to the danger point of 42° C (108° C) or when evaporative cooling is poor because of high air humidity, it is necessary to immerse the victim in a bath of water or under a shower. Usually there is no opportunity of taking accurate core temperature readings and assessment of the degree of hyperthermia has to be based on the state of consciousness and on whether the subject is still sweating.

In theory, cold water should be the most efficient treatment because it creates the greatest thermal gradient. In practice, contact of the skin with cold water causes massive discharge of cutaneous cold receptors, which activates heat retention outflows from the hypothalamus including profound cutaneous vasoconstriction. The massive fall in skin blood flow prevents effective heat loss. This can lead to core temperature rising further to a critical value as stored tissue heat enters the bloodstream, before the central thermoreceptors override the peripheral input. It is, therefore, safer and more efficient to use water that is tepid or around room temperature than that typically coming from a cold water supply.

The other effective alternative would be to create a thermal gradient so large that there will be rapid heat loss even in the absence of skin blood flow, by immersion in an ice–water mixture. This strategy is often recommended for treatment of individuals whose internal temperatures are critically high and who are unconscious as a result. In awake people, on the other hand, sudden whole-body immersion in ice water is too painful for it to be the method of choice.

## Tissue damage due to fluid depletion

Plasma volume depletion equivalent to reduction of total blood volume by 1.5 l or more is sufficient to reduce mean blood pressure even when sympathetic drive is maximal. In these circumstances, the consequent fall in tissue perfusion may have deleterious outcomes unless effective fluid replacement is achieved within 1–2 h. The problems occur mainly in regions of the circulation where microcirculatory counter-current exchange leads to local hypoxia (see Chapter 5, p. 58). In the kidney, the fall in medullary blood flow can cause necrotic damage to the loops of Henle and the collecting ducts, resulting in loss of urinary concentrating power and further fluid loss. In the small intestine, the fall in perfusion of the villi can result in sloughing of the villar epithelium, leading to exposure of the underlying tissue to intestinal proteolytic enzymes and to potential entry into the bloodstream of Gram-negative bacteria that are normally restricted to the gut lumen.

If blood pressure is low enough to prevent effective capillary perfusion through some areas of peripheral tissues, then blood cells begin to fall out of suspension and form clumps within the downstream venules (see Chapter 5, p. 60). Once this has occurred, even restoration of blood volume sufficient to reduce peripheral resistance to normal may not restore effective perfusion in these areas, because the venular cell clumps create a resistance sufficient to redirect blood flow to other, lower resistance, regions of the tissue.

## Drug-induced hyperthermia

The 3,4-methylenedioxymethamphetamine molecule, commonly known as ecstasy, is widely used as a recreational drug and has been the cause of a number of deaths due to hyperthermia. Ecstasy has several pharmacological properties that collectively predispose to elevated core temperature (Mills et al 2004). First, it increases central sympathetic drive, with resulting cutaneous vasoconstriction. Second, it acts in a variety of tissues to stimulate uncoupling proteins. These uncouple mitochondrial respiration from ATP synthesis and so generate additional metabolic heat. Third, it appears to act on amine-receptive synapses in the hypothalamus to reset the central thermostat to a higher operating point.

Given this combination of excess heat production and reduced capacity for heat loss, it is not surprising that ecstasy can cause dangerous rises in core temperature in individuals who are also exercising. The risk is even greater for regular rather than for casual ecstasy users, since chronic ingestion upregulates secretion of thyroid hormones and, therefore, elevates basal metabolic rate and heat production.

## Exertional rhabdomyolysis

A small number of people have a defect in the RYR1 gene that encodes calcium channels in skeletal muscle sarcoplasmic reticulum. This can under some conditions result in excessive calcium entry to the sarcomeres during contraction and, therefore, more muscle heat production than normal. When these individuals undertake prolonged exercise, their core temperatures can rise to dangerous levels and the even greater elevation of local temperature in exercising muscles results in muscle cell breakdown (*rhabdomyolysis*). Even with adequate reversal of the hyperthermia, this situation can have fatal consequences, as the large amounts of liberated intracellular potassium impair cardiac rhythm and the liberated myoglobin is filtered in the kidney and may occlude the renal tubules, leading to acute renal failure.

Rhabdomyolysis has as well been reported as a consequence of ecstasy intoxication, presumably in individuals with similar genotypic predispositions. Because the abnormal calcium channel function appears to only occur during prolonged muscle activation, short bouts of even intense exercise do not generate excessive heat and so are not associated with risk of hyperthermic damage (Muldoon et al 2004).

## SUDDEN CARDIAC DEATH

Occasionally, an apparently normal young individual collapses and dies during exercise because the heart stops beating. This so-called *sudden cardiac death* is extremely rare (of the order of one individual per 50 000 per year), so it is unlikely to occur in any exercise-related research study, but such a serious event has to be borne in mind as a remote possibility. By definition, sudden cardiac death in athletes does not involve overt cardiac disease processes, but it obviously must involve some abnormality of cardiac function that is triggered or exacerbated by exercise.

There are two main causes of sudden cardiac death (Catanzaro et al 2006, Corrado et al 2006). One is a genetically determined type of cardiac muscle cell membrane abnormality (*hypertrophic cardiomyopathy*), characterized by increased capacity to generate arrhythmias. The second is developmental abnormality of the coronary arteries. The left and right coronary arteries normally arise from the left and right sides of the aortic sinus respectively and run from there to the left and right myocardium. Occasionally, however, both arteries arise from the same side of the aortic sinus and so one must travel between the aorta and the pulmonary artery in order to reach the appropriate side of the heart. When cardiac output rises during exercise, aorta and pulmonary arteries become distended and the aberrant coronary artery may be compressed, resulting in hypoxia to that side of the heart.

Much debate has gone on as to whether routine screening programmes should be put in place to exclude individuals with one of these abnormalities from participating in sport (Corrado et al 2006). In practice, this would be extremely difficult and the benefits would be uncertain. Retrospective analysis indicates that only a minority of individuals who sustain sudden cardiac death during exercise have any suggestive signs, including identifiable ECG abnormalities. Finding those at risk would, therefore, require complex and expensive investigations, with, even then, no guarantee that all such individuals would be identified. Against this approach is the certainty that participation in sports programmes has proven advantages for health in general and that many people involved in sports would be likely to choose to continue their involvement in spite of a known risk.

On balance, a sensible approach seems to be as follows. Identify by careful screening the people at obvious risk (history of fainting or dizziness, ECG evidence of atrial fibrillation, ventricular extrasystoles or ischaemia) and exclude them from experimental exercise studies. Ensure that individuals in this category are investigated further before being accepted into competitive sports programmes. But also recognize that a tiny number of unidentifiable people will remain at risk and in whom it is entirely uncertain whether they might die as a result of exercise.

## Key points

Static and resistive exercise modalities tend to increase intrathoracic pressure. In erect subjects, the resulting fall in cardiac filling can reduce blood pressure and cerebral perfusion sufficiently to cause loss of consciousness.

The plasma volume depletion associated with sweat production during exercise, especially under ambient conditions of high relative humidity and high temperature, can lead to collapse due to reduced cerebral perfusion.

When evaporative heat loss is obstructed by insulative clothing, core temperature can rise rapidly during exercise to levels that may be fatal.

In treating athletes who have collapsed because of either heat-induced fluid loss or hyperthermia, it is important to remember that body temperature may continue to rise after exercise ceases as metabolic heat diffuses out of previously active muscles.

A very small percentage of individuals possess congenital abnormalities that predispose them to adverse effects of exercise. Among these are muscle defects that cause excessive heat production and cardiac abnormalities that can result in fatal arrhythmias.

## References

Catanzaro JN, Makaryus AN, Catanese C 2006 Sudden cardiac death associated with an extremely rare coronary anomaly of the left and right coronary arteries arising exclusively from the posterior (noncoronary) sinus of Valsalva. Clinical Cardiology 28: 542–544.

Corrado D, Basso C, Pavei A et al 2006 Trends in sudden cardiovascular death in young competitive athletes after implementation of a preparticipation screening program. Journal of the American Medical Association 296: 1593–1601.

Hernandez JP, Franke WD 2004 Age- and fitness-related differences in limb venous compliance do not affect tolerance to maximal lower body negative pressure in men and women. Journal of Applied Physiology 97: 925–929.

Muldoon S, Deuster P, Brandom B, Bunger R 2004 Is there a link between malignant hyperthermia and exertional heat illness? Exercise and Sport Science Reviews 32: 174–179.

Mills EM, Rusyniak DE, Sprague JE 2004 The role of the sympathetic nervous system and uncoupling proteins in the thermogenesis induced by 3,4-methylenedioxymethamphetamine. Journal of Molecular Medicine 82: 787–799.

**Questions for revision**

- Describe the normal cardiovascular response to a sustained increase in intrathoracic pressure.

- Why might a weight lifter be more likely to faint during competition than during training?

- Define and distinguish heat exhaustion and heat stroke.

- In dealing with an athlete who collapses with a core temperature of 41° C (106° F), why is it important to reduce core temperature as quickly as possible and how can this best be achieved?

- What are the main causes of sudden cardiac death in athletes?

# Chapter 11

# Cardiovascular adaptations to chronic exercise

## CHAPTER CONTENTS

### After reading this chapter, you should:

- appreciate the changes in blood volume and cardiovascular structure and function that follow dynamic physical training
- know the approximate extent to which these changes alter capacity for aerobic work
- understand the roles for chronic exercise in treatment of common cardiovascular disease states

Athletic training oriented to a particular type of dynamic exercise has the effect of modifying muscle fibre metabolism towards pathways that suit that exercise modality. However, these metabolic adaptations can confer only little or no advantage on exercise performance without concurrent enhancement of the circulatory support of muscle oxygen consumption by increased blood delivery. The concept of physical fitness is, therefore, one centred on cardiovascular adaptation so as to increase cardiac output to values greater than those achievable in the pre-training state – in other words, to increase cardiac reserve.

From the issues discussed in previous chapters it will be clear that one's capacity to elevate cardiac output could be improved by increasing blood volume, by reducing resting heart rate (that is, increasing heart rate reserve) or by increasing stroke volume. It should also be remembered that cardiovascular capacity to service muscle metabolism is normally limited by the simultaneous thermoregulatory demands. Therefore, exercise capacity will be increased by minimizing hyperthermia and the associated encroachments on muscle blood flow and plasma volume that result from cutaneous vasodilation and sweating.

All of these adaptations occur, but they have very different timecourses. An initial increase in work capacity linked to increased cardiac reserve occurs over a matter of several weeks' training, but the achievable cardiac output continues to rise over the succeeding months so that with any given training schedule, peak performance, as determined by cardiovascular efficiency, will not be reached until after around 9–12 months (Fig. 11.1).

## BLOOD-VOLUME ADAPTATIONS

### Plasma volume

Training induces a maintained elevation of plasma volume by of the order of 10%; that is evident after even a single bout of dynamic training. The initial volume increase involves retention of sodium and water only, secondary to increased numbers of aldosterone receptors in the distal tubule. Over 2–3 days' training, there is an associated rise in circulating albumin that restores plasma oncotic pressure to normal.

The signals that transduce these changes have not been identified with certainty. However, it seems likely that activation of the aldosterone pathway is triggered by the rise in plasma potassium caused by muscle activation, while hepatic albumin synthesis is probably stimulated by the cortisol release that accompanies dynamic activity.

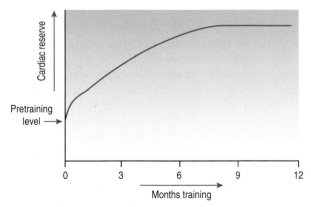

**Figure 11.1** Representation of the timecourse of increase in maximum cardiac output over a 12-month period of dynamic exercise training. Note the small, initial rise due primarily to blood-volume expansion, followed by several months' progressive rise that involves further cardiac adaptations and peripheral vascular changes.

## Red cell volume

The changes in plasma volume described above produce an initial fall in haematocrit, but with continued training there is, over the ensuing several weeks, increased erythropoiesis that restores the concentration of red cells to its previous level. The likely stimulus for increased red cell production is the recurrent renal medullary hypoxia associated with renal sympathetic activation, which results in release of erythropoietin from medullary tubule cells.

Collectively, the changes in blood volume constitute the major cause of the rise in cardiac reserve that is seen over the first 3–4 weeks of training (Fig. 11.1). As we shall see below, increased heart rate reserve also has a role during this period.

## CARDIAC ADAPTATIONS

### Heart rate reserve

Resting heart rate often begins to fall after the first few sessions of regular dynamic exercise and may be around 10 beats/min lower than the pre-training value after 2 weeks of training (Murray et al 2006). This confers an immediate advantage on exercise capacity, since it increases heart rate reserve. A 20 year old with a resting heart rate of 70 beats/min can theoretically increase cardiac output by (200–70/70) or 1.85-fold by tachycardia alone: with a resting heart rate of 60 beats/min this increase becomes (200–60/60) or 2.33-fold. Thus, in order to undertake any given submaximal workload, the trained individual needs only to increase heart rate (and, therefore, cardiac workload) by (1.85/2.33) or 80% of the amount needed before training.

This early bradycardia is at least mainly a reflex result of the blood volume expansion induced by training, sensed as increased atrial filling by low-pressure baroreceptors and as increased stroke volume by high-pressure baroreceptors. A second contributing factor may be the reduction of sympathetic drive that results from repetitive central command (see Vascular adaptations, below). The magnitude of the early bradycardia does not appear to be affected greatly by training intensity and its relatively small magnitude has only a limited effect on work capacity, as shown by the calculations in the previous paragraph.

In individuals who train intensively for prolonged periods, much greater degrees of bradycardia develop due to increased vagal tone, such that resting heart rate may be as low as 35 beats/min. This obviously confers a far larger cardiac reserve, with the 20-year-old athlete being theoretically able to increase his cardiac output by (200–35/35) or 4.7-fold using tachycardia alone, and reducing his cardiac workload for a given submaximal work intensity to (1.85/4.7) or 40% of that in an untrained age-matched individual.

This more dramatic bradycardic effect of prolonged training is secondary to structural adaptation of the heart (see Cardiac hypertrophy, below).

During incremental dynamic exercise, it has been found that many trained athletes do not produce linear increases in heart rate up to their age-limited maximum. Instead, the slope of the heart rate/work curve flattens at around 85% $\dot{V}O_{2max}$ (Lepretre et al 2005). Since this workload corresponds approximately to the anaerobic threshold, the heart rate deflection point has been adopted in a number of centres as an easy, non-invasive monitor for setting training workloads. It has also been suggested that the deflection infers some advantage on athletes by allowing greater utilization of their capacity to increase cardiac output by increasing stroke volume, although no firm evidence base for this exists. Regardless of whether or not the phenomenon has a value, the mechanisms that underlie it are unknown, and its usefulness as a training aid is limited by its variable occurrence even in trained athletes.

## Cardiac hypertrophy

Like skeletal muscle, the myocardium responds to chronically increased workload by muscle cell growth, resulting in what is traditionally known as the 'athlete's heart' (Iglesias Cubero et al 2000). As in skeletal muscle, the pattern of growth varies depending on whether the increased work is dynamic or resistive. Increased ventricular filling (increased *preload*), with no change in outflow resistance, results in moderately thickened muscle around an enlarged ventricular chamber (*eccentric hypertrophy*). By contrast, increased resistance to outflow (increased *afterload*) due, for instance, to increased peripheral resistance, leads to a markedly thickened ventricular wall with no alteration of chamber size (*concentric hypertrophy*) (Fig. 11.2).

Chronic dynamic exercise exerts both of these effects on the heart; the increased preload, because of increased venous return, and the increased afterload, because of the pressor response to central command. Not surprisingly, therefore, the initial structural adaptations to dynamic training involve

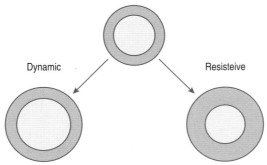

Dynamic

Resisteive

**Figure 11.2** Hypertrophic changes of the ventricular myocardium in response to dynamic and resistive training. Dynamic training results in increased chamber size as well as wall thickening, while resistive training preferentially increases wall thickness with little or no increase in chamber size.

elements of both types of hypertrophy. In the right heart, little or no afterload increase takes place because the pulmonary vasculature is exempted from sympathetic vasoconstrictor influences and, in fact, pulmonary vascular resistance falls during exercise due to better ventilation/perfusion matching (see Chapter 8, p. 95). The right ventricle, therefore, shows uncomplicated eccentric hypertrophy. On the left side, however, there are increases in both preload and afterload, which induces some degree of concentric hypertrophy and limits the expansion of left ventricular chamber size until after around 6–9 months training. Thus, the full benefits of cardiac adaptation, in terms of increased stroke volume, are not evident until after this period.

From the preceding discussion, it should be obvious that static exercise has far less effect than dynamic exercise on resting stroke volume and heart rate, because it precludes ventricular chamber enlargement. This has some significance for the training of rowers, in whom massive elevation of cardiac reserve is essential for good performance, but who also experience large rises in afterload during the catch phase of the stroke. Training programmes, therefore, should not involve rowing alone, but include additional dynamic exercises devoid of resistive components.

The cardiac changes seen in concentric hypertrophy also bear consideration in relation to the implications for endocardial pressure. During contraction, the pressure within the ventricular wall rises with wall thickness, according to Laplace's law, with the greatest pressure being in the endocardial layer. This means that coronary perfusion of the endocardium becomes less efficient as wall thickness rises, with greater potential for endocardial hypoxia and initiation of arrhythmias.

The progressive bradycardia that accompanies prolonged training tracks the development of ventricular hypertrophy and stroke volume increase. It is probably, therefore, at least partly due to baroreflex withdrawal of sinoatrial sympathetic drive and increased vagal drive, secondary to stroke volume increase. In addition, however, some evidence suggests that long periods of neurally induced bradycardia may result in changes in intrinsic sinoatrial membrane channel cycling, with resetting of the basic pacemaker potential slope to a lower gradient.

## VASCULAR ADAPTATIONS

The resting bradycardia associated with training is accompanied by reduced total peripheral resistance. In studies that have tracked previously sedentary subjects through a training programme, the fall in peripheral resistance has been seen to cause a fall in mean resting blood pressure of up to around 10 mmHg (Murray et al 2006). There is, however, considerable variation between individuals in the magnitude of the effect and the available data suggest that little or no further effect on pressure occurs in highly trained athletes than is seen with moderately improved fitness. The fall in peripheral resistance that follows training may involve several mechanisms.

## Sympathetic drive

In view of the apparent reduction in sympathetic vasomotor tone following acute exercise (see Chapter 7, p. 79) and the likely baroreflex effects of expanded blood volume, it might be expected that resting sympathetic drive would be reduced following training. In fact, microneurographic studies of action potential frequency in sympathetic nerve filaments provide no support for this, although for technical reasons these studies use muscle nerves and so give no information on the behaviour of, for example, splanchnic vasomotor control (Alvarez et al 2005).

There is, by contrast, good evidence that training reduces pressor responses to stimuli that cause sympathetic activation. Trained individuals have been found to exhibit less blood pressure rise in response to some laboratory stressors such as mental arithmetic and also to have less pronounced pressor responses to given increments of exercise. These changes may be due to reduced gain in the hindbrain responses to central command and could involve endorphin release (see Chapter 7, p. 85). Desensitization of peripheral metaboreceptors and limb mechanoreceptors may also be involved. In terms of training-mediated effects on performance, damping of sympathetic drive may be beneficial in allowing greater increments of muscle blood flow in response to local dilator factors during muscle activation (see Chapter 6, p. 72).

## Endothelial function

Training is associated with increased endothelium-dependent dilator capacity, as indicated by the magnitudes of responses to reactive hyperaemia (see Chapter 6, p. 66) and by resting plasma levels of nitric oxide (NO). One possible mechanism is that the increased endothelial turnover caused by repetitive exercise-induced shear stress results in a systemic endothelial lining with a younger mean cell age that, therefore, has greater secretory capacity. There is evidence that endothelial function is affected preferentially in the vascular beds of those muscles that have been repetitively exercised (Thijssen et al 2005), so the extent of peripheral resistance reduction is likely to correlate with the proportion of the whole-body musculature that is used. This is an issue that needs to be considered when designing training programmes for patients with limited mobility.

## Angiogenesis

With prolonged dynamic training, local release of vascular endothelial growth factor and other growth factors leads to sprouting of new capillaries and arterioles in the active skeletal muscles and the myocardium. Appearance of these new vessels necessarily lowers regional vascular resistance, as well as reducing the distance for diffusion of nutrients and metabolites between blood stream and cells. Much less effect on vascular resistance is seen with static or intense resistive training, since the capillary density in type IIb glycolytic muscle is considerably sparser than in oxidative muscles.

## Arterial remodelling

It is not clear whether the angiogenic responses of the microcirculation to vascular growth factors are associated also with increased growth of large conducting arteries. If this occurred, it would cause a small but significant reduction in total peripheral resistance. To my knowledge, data are available only for the coronary vasculature. Isolated post-mortem findings have reported enlarged coronary arteries in elite athletes, but imaging studies of living athletes has not provided evidence that even intense training has an effect on resting diameters of the major coronary vessels.

## THERMOREGULATORY ADAPTATIONS

Chronic exposure to either a hot external environment or to repetitive episodes of increased internal heat production, as occurs during dynamic exercise, results in the hypothalamic thermostat becoming more sensitive to inputs from central (blood) heat detectors. Compensatory heat loss processes are, therefore, activated with less displacement of core temperature from the set point, and cutaneous vasodilation and sweat secretion begin after shorter latency during an exercise bout. This reduces the amount of metabolic heat trapped in the body and so reduces the absolute rise in body temperature at any given workload. As well, the reduced volume of sweat required for heat loss reduces the need for cutaneous hyperaemia and so makes more blood flow available for muscle perfusion.

This is a further rapid thermoregulatory adaptation to result from the increased aldosterone secretion that follows exercise-induced hyperkalaemia (see above, p. 130). As in the renal tubules, aldosterone acts on sweat ducts to reabsorb sodium. In the presence of greater numbers of aldosterone receptors, therefore, the sodium content of sweat falls dramatically, from around 50 mmol/L in a sedentary exercising subject to around 5 mmol/L in a trained subject. Thus, although total water loss in sweat may rise in the trained individual, due to the greater amount of muscle work undertaken, plasma and extracellular fluid osmolality are maintained far more efficiently.

Figure 11.3 summarizes the adaptive responses to dynamic training, as discussed above.

## GENDER DIFFERENCES

Closely similar effects of training are seen in men and women with respect to fitness, although the absolute effect of training is limited in women by their smaller heart size, in a similar way to their lower limit to acute exercise.

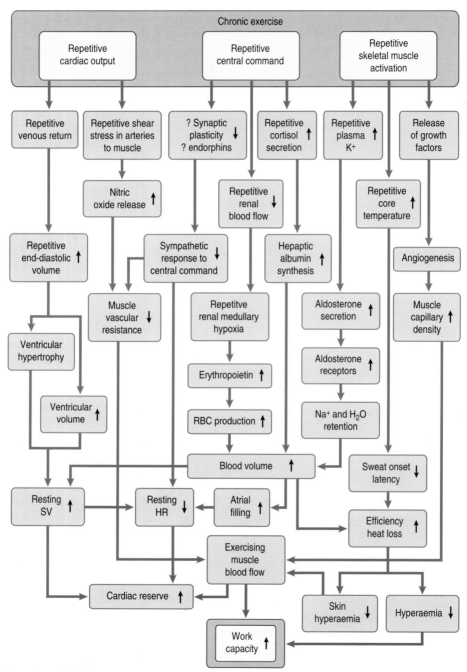

**Figure 11.3** The causes and results of adaptive cardiovascular responses to chronic dynamic exercise that lead to increased physical fitness.

Some investigators have reported that women are less able than men to produce cardiac hypertrophy in response to increased preload and have suggested that peripheral vascular adaptations may play a greater part than in men. However, these conclusions may have been distorted by the smaller initial heart size in women: the consensus of opinion now is that equivalent cardiac changes proportionate to heart mass occur in both sexes (Whyte et al 2004).

## DETRAINING

The adaptive cardiovascular effects of training are lost if training ceases over timecourses that broadly reflect the times taken for their onset. Thus, plasma volume falls within a few days and whole blood volume over 2–3 weeks, with parallel reduction in maximum cardiac output. The increases in endothelial dilator capacity are also completely reversed by 2 weeks after training stops. The effect on achievable workload ($\dot{V}O_{2max}$) of short-term (of the order of weeks) training is, therefore, completely lost again within a matter of weeks, a fact that needs to be considered in relation to the potential long-term benefits of cardiac rehabilitation programmes.

After long-term (many months) training, by contrast, $\dot{V}O_{2max}$ falls more gradually, as the reversals of muscle angiogenesis and cardiac hypertrophy take place over the order of months. Notwithstanding, there is some evidence that, in athletes who have trained for many years, some cardiac hypertrophy may persist permanently.

## ROLE OF EXERCISE IN CARDIOVASCULAR THERAPY

### Atherosclerosis as the main cause of cardiovascular disability

Together with cancer, cardiovascular disease represents the largest cause of mortality in Western societies. Almost all cases of death or incapacitation of cardiovascular origin are caused by atherosclerosis, a pathological process that involves fatty precipitates (*atheromatous plaques*) being deposited in large arteries at sites of endothelial damage. These plaques partially obstruct the arterial lumen, reducing nutritional blood flow. They may also be dislodged into the bloodstream as *thrombi,* where they travel to more distal sites and block the blood supply to areas of peripheral tissues, a process termed *infarction.*

### Common sites of atherosclerotic damage

The tissues most sensitive to this local deprivation of flow are those with the greatest continuous need for oxygen – the myocardium and the brain. So the characteristic results of atheromatous thrombus formation are myocardial infarctions or *heart attacks,* and cerebral infarctions or *strokes.* The effect of less severe restriction of blood flow due to atherosclerotic luminal narrowing is most usually seen as chest pain when acidic metabolites accumulate in an area of the myocardium where coronary perfusion is reduced, causing stimulation of chemosensitive nerve endings. This type of pain caused by inadequate local blood flow is known as *angina*.

Plaques can also partially occlude the large arteries that supply the legs. The consequences of this reflect the fact that progressively smaller arteries contribute progressively more to regional vascular resistance. Thus, when there is moderate thrombotic obstruction to flow in the femoral or iliac arteries, blood flow to the legs is usually normal at rest, but the usual functional hyperaemia associated with exercise is impaired. This results in accumulation of acidic metabolites in the working muscle, with development of anginal leg pain after a short period of walking that makes the patient stop. The latency of onset of pain is related to the workload and, typically, the patient is able, after a short rest, to repeat a similar amount of exercise before the pain recurs. This pattern of periodic exercise-induced pain is termed *intermittent claudication*. When the same degree of thrombotic blockage occurs in one of the smaller, more distal arteries, there is reduced blood flow at rest, resulting in continual leg pain and ischaemic tissue damage (*gangrene*).

## Hypertension predisposes to atherosclerosis

Long-term studies of the incidence of cardiovascular disease in large populations (*epidemiological studies*) have shown that atherosclerosis is more common in people who have relatively high blood pressures. The presence of high resting blood pressure (*hypertension*) has, therefore, become an independent predictive marker for heart attacks and strokes. Although guidelines vary across the world, the most common current threshold for hypertension is a resting blood pressure that is consistently higher than 140/90 mmHg. With this threshold, over 20% of all adults in Western societies are classified as hypertensive and, therefore, by definition require some sort of treatment – most usually pharmacological – in order to reduce their blood pressures.

The epidemiological evidence suggests that incidence of atherosclerosis is correlated with absolute blood pressure over the entire range of pressures that exist in man so, in theory, the lower the pressure, the less likely an individual is to sustain an adverse event. By this criterion, it would be advantageous to amend the current guidelines so as to reduce the pressure threshold for hypertension. However, the distribution of blood pressures in the community means that even lowering the threshold by 1 mmHg would result in an additional 1% of the population being classified as abnormal. Any benefits from reduced incidence of infarcts would have to be balanced against the massively increased costs of patient management. As well, there would be significant ethical questions about arbitrary classification of currently healthy individuals as patients and prescribing them drugs that have predictable side effects.

The increased risk of cardiovascular events associated with hypertension is probably related to the rapid increase in vessel wall tension as transmural pressure rises, in line with Laplace's law (see Chapter 5, p. 52), since increased tension will facilitate breakdown of the endothelial barrier at sites of pre-existing cell damage and so aid plaque formation. High intravascular pressure will also, by increasing blood flow velocity, increase marginal shear stress in large arteries and facilitate dislodgement of pre-existing plaques. In addition, the increased cardiac afterload due to hypertension will lead to concentric hypertrophy of the left ventricle. This lowers coronary capillary density and increases systolic endocardial compression, reducing functional cardiac reserve and predisposing the heart to hypoxic damage.

## Case history

A 58-year-old man, John J., was considering discontinuing his gym membership because his left calf ached when he exercised on the treadmill. He took up weight training instead, but 2 months later was still having pain during any prolonged exercise that required lower limb contractions. He was able to walk about 200 m without trouble, but after that his left leg ached so much that he had to stop. After a few minutes rest, he could walk the same distance again before the pain recurred.

In the exercise lab, measurements of blood flow were made in each of his calves, at rest and immediately after moderate cycle exercise (60 rpm, 80 W) until onset of pain (approx. 1 min). In his left and right legs respectively, resting flows were 2.4 and 2.6 ml/min/100 ml tissue and exercise flows were 8 and 18 ml/min/100 ml tissue.

## Discussion

John's problem is a typical case of intermittent claudication owing to structural narrowing of the artery supplying his left lower leg. The cause cannot be ascertained without clinical investigations, but could involve atherosclerosis or connective tissue disease. Smoking is a very common risk factor.

Chronic limb pain associated with exercise is almost always due to chemoreceptor activation by accumulated muscle metabolites, implying a local increase in vascular resistance that limits muscle perfusion. John's absence of pain except during exercise indicated that his leg blood flow was sufficient to service muscle metabolism at rest. This was confirmed by the similar and normal blood flow data recorded from both legs. During dynamic exercise, by contrast, blood flow rose sixfold in the right leg, but only threefold in the left.

This pattern of normal flow at rest and impaired flow under circumstances of functional hyperaemia is characteristic of localized constriction in a large conducting artery. Increased resistance in the microcirculation, by contrast, would be expected to impair tissue perfusion more or less independent of nutritional demand.

## Chronic exercise has several anti-atherogenic effects

From consideration of these causal factors, chronic dynamic exercise can be seen to have several effects that potentially help prevent or reverse atherosclerosis-related cardiovascular changes. Improved endothelial cell function will reduce the susceptibility of the endothelium to traumatic or chemical damage. Increased endothelial dilator capacity and increased muscle capillary density will reduce peripheral resistance and, together with reduced sympathetic responses to arousal, will lower pressor responses to a variety of stimuli. This pressure reduction, the relative bradycardia induced by training and the conversion of concentric cardiac hypertrophy to eccentric hypertrophy will all reduce cardiac workload. Finally, the concomitant increase in coronary capillary density will help reduce any local myocardial ischaemia produced by atheromatous blockage. Figure 11.4 summarizes these therapeutic effects of training.

## Exercise in cardiac rehabilitation

Following myocardial infarction the affected region of the myocardium may, depending on the degree of hypoxia, consist of dead muscle cells or contain at least some cells that can recover their contractile function. In either situation, chronic exercise provides a valuable stimulus to improvement of cardiac contractility. In the case of hypoxic but living myocardial tissue, exercise increases coronary perfusion by elevating blood pressure and by stimulating angiogenesis. Where an area of myocardium is dead, then the angiogenic effect of exercise helps to increase perfusion of the remaining myocardium. In both cases, the multiple consequences of training that reduce cardiac afterload (Fig. 11.4) will optimize resting cardiac function and enhance cardiac reserve.

Typical exercise sessions in cardiac rehabilitation settings last for around 30 min and include a variety of modalities spanning dynamic and resistive exercises. Although cardiovascular benefits can be predicted to accrue predominantly from the dynamic components, providing a range of exercises is valuable in maintaining patient motivation and caters for individuals who may have limited mobility.

Despite the clear theoretical benefits of exercise programmes in aiding recovery from cardiac infarcts, and general agreement that they are effective, very little objective data exist concerning the advantages and limitations of different exercise intensities or programme durations. Part of the problem is the difficulty in quantifying exercise performance in this patient group. At least initially, most are unable to work at more than around 20% of their calculated maximum work capacity because of their coronary impairment. In addition, almost all patients are routinely prescribed $\beta$-adrenoceptor antagonists to limit their cardiac workload. They are consequently not able to produce normal work-intensity-related tachycardia. Under these

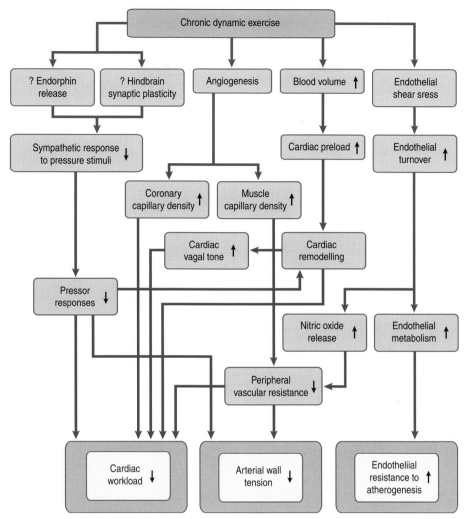

**Figure 11.4** The effects of chronic dynamic exercise on factors that predispose to atherosclerosis-related cardiovascular events.

circumstances it is necessary to make a number of assumptions about the workloads undertaken, based primarily on the patients' subjective perceptions of how hard they are working (American Association of Cardiovascular and Pulmonary Rehabilitation 2006). Well-designed research would be extremely helpful in ascertaining how these rehabilitation strategies can be optimized and how the benefits that accrue can be maintained after patients complete a supervised programme.

## References

Alvarez GE, Halliwill JR, Ballard TP, Beske SD, Davy KP 2005 Sympathetic neural regulation in endurance-trained humans: fitness vs. fatness. Journal of Applied Physiology 98: 498–502.

American Association of Cardiovascular and Pulmonary Rehabilitation 2006 AACVPR Cardiac Rehabilitation Resource Manual. Human Kinetics, Champaign, IL.

Iglesias Cubero G, Batalla A, Rodriguez Reguero JJ et al 2000 Left ventricular mass index and sports: the influence of different sports activities and arterial blood pressure. International Journal of Cardiology 75: 261–265.

Lepretre P-M, Foster C, Koralsztein J-P, Billat VL 2005 Heart rate deflection point as a strategy to defend stroke volume during incremental exercise. Journal of Applied Physiology 98: 1660–1665.

Murray Á, Delaney T, Bell C 2006 Rapid onset and offset of circulatory adaptations to exercise training in men. Journal of Human Hypertension 20: 193–200.

Thijssen DH, Heesterbeek P, van Kuppevelt DJ, Duysens J, Hopman MT 2005 Local vascular adaptations after hybrid training in spinal cord-injured subjects. Medicine and Science of Sports and Exercise 37: 1112–1118.

Whyte GP, George K, Sharma S et al 2004 The upper limit of physiological cardiac hypertrophy in elite male and female athletes: the British experience. European Journal of Applied Physiology 92: 592–597.

## Questions for revision

- List the main parameters that contribute to the increased capacity for maximal cardiac output during a programme of dynamic exercise training.

- Define eccentric and concentric cardiac hypertrophy. Which type of hypertrophy occurs in response to dynamic exercise training?

- What theromoregulatory adaptations occur in response to regular physical activity?

- Define intermittent claudication and write notes on its effects.

- Discuss the ways in which regular exercise may reduce the risk of atherosclerotic vascular disease.

# Chapter **12**

# Effects of high altitude

## CHAPTER CONTENTS

### After reading this chapter, you should:

- understand the acute and chronic effects of high altitude on exercise capacity
- appreciate the rationale for training at altitude
- comprehend the implications of this for optimizing exercise performance
- appreciate how exposure to high altitude may disrupt normal physiological homeostasis

## ALTITUDE AND OXYGEN TRANSPORT

### Effects of altitude on plasma oxygen uptake

The standard atmospheric pressure of 760 mmHg (101 kPa) at sea level reflects the weight exerted by the gas molecules that make up the air, under gravitational force. As one ascends from sea level, the air becomes progressively less compressed and so the constituent gas molecules become less tightly packed. In consequence, a given volume of inspired air contains fewer molecules of all gases, including oxygen. The relationship between altitude and atmospheric pressure is not a strictly linear one because the air volume increases in 3 dimensions but, in rough terms, pressure falls by around 100 mmHg for every 1000 m (3300 ft) of ascent up to 3000 m (10 000 ft) (Fig. 12.1).

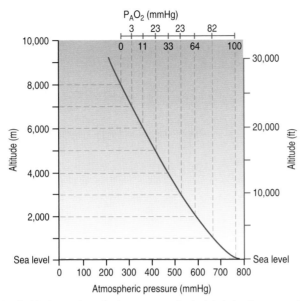

**Figure 12.1** Effects of altitude on atmospheric pressure and calculated alveolar oxygen tension ($P_AO_2$). $P_AO_2$ values have been estimated as ([21%.$P_{atmos}$–47] – 50) and represent the theoretical values that result from atmospheric pressure alone, disregarding any physiological compensations that occur. Note that in this theoretical situation $P_AO_2$ falls to zero at an altitude of 8000 m (26 000 ft) although, with acclimation, numerous individuals have climbed to the summit of Mt Everest at 8843 m (29 000 ft).

The absolute change in oxygen availability imposed by a given ascent can be calculated easily. Since oxygen represents 21% of normal air, the partial pressure of oxygen ($PO_2$) at sea level is (21%.760) or 160 mmHg. Once inspired, the air becomes saturated with water vapour (partial pressure 47 mmHg) so that the total gas pressure is reduced to 713 mmHg and $PO_2$ falls to (21%.713) or 150 mmHg. In the alveoli, the oxygen is diluted further by approximately 50 mmHg, due primarily to the presence of carbon dioxide, resulting in a local $PO_2$ ($P_AO_2$) of around 100 mmHg: at equilibrium with the plasma, arterial $PO_2$ ($PaO_2$) is, therefore, usually also around 100 mmHg.

At an atmospheric pressure of 560 mmHg, which corresponds to an altitude of around 2300 m (7600 ft) or just higher than Mexico City, $P_AO_2$ can be estimated to be around 60 mmHg (21%.[560–47] – 50). Many of the major ski resorts like Aspen and Zermatt involve slopes at heights in excess of 3500 m (11 000 ft), where atmospheric pressure is 500 mmHg and so $P_AO_2$ will be around (21%. [500–47] – 50) or 45 mmHg, while permanent settlements in the Himalayas and Andes are found as high as 5000 m (17 500 ft) where atmospheric pressure is only 390 mmHg and calculated $P_AO_2$ is around 25 mmHg.

## Effects of altitude on oxygen carriage

Because of the sigmoid shape of the haemoglobin dissociation curve, the falls in $PaO_2$ associated with acute exposure to altitudes up to around 2000 m

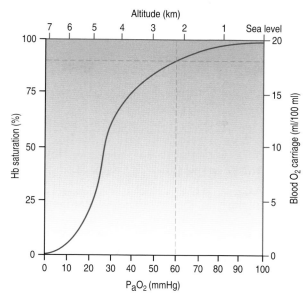

**Figure 12.2** Relationship between altitude, arterial oxygen tension (PaO$_2$), haemoglobin saturation and blood oxygen carriage. Note that at the altitude where PaO$_2$ reaches the threshold for peripheral hypoxia receptor activation (60 mmHg) blood oxygen carriage is reduced only marginally from the sea level value.

(6700 ft) cause only a slight reduction in haemoglobin saturation (Fig. 12.2) and so do not reduce oxygen delivery at rest. During exercise, however, the combination of reduced binding and reduced pulmonary capillary transit time leads to a greater degree of desaturation that is proportional both to altitude and to cardiac output. Thus, the threshold altitude for oxygen limitation of maximum exercise in sedentary individuals is typically around 1500 m (5000 ft), but, in trained athletes with substantially greater cardiac outputs, maximum work capacity begins to fall at much lower altitudes (Johnson et al 1994). In the only Summer Olympics held at a significant altitude, in Mexico City in 1968, winning times for all track events longer than 800 m were well above the existing records.

## COMPENSATION FOR HYPOXIA

### Respiratory stimulation

The reduced oxygen carriage associated with moderate altitude results in more rapid fatigue during exercise, but no respiratory compensation occurs because ventilation is still driven by the central chemoreceptors. These respond to rises in local proton concentration (that is, reduced pH) secondary to arterial carbon dioxide diffusing into the hindbrain, but are insensitive to hypoxia. The peripheral chemoreceptors responsible for monitoring arterial oxygen status are triggered only when PaO$_2$ falls to around

60 mmHg which, as we saw earlier (p. 145), corresponds to an approximate altitude of 2300 m or 7600 ft. At or above this height, chemoreceptor stimulation initiates increased minute ventilation the magnitude of which depends both on the initial $PaO_2$ and on whether increased ventilation is able to restore $PaO_2$ to a value above 60 mmHg.

This acute ventilatory compensation for hypoxia occurs very rapidly, but is itself able to produce only a moderate improvement in oxygen availability. The reason is that increased ventilation necessarily results in carbon dioxide being blown off at a greater rate than before, leading to a fall in arterial carbon dioxide ($PaCO_2$) (*hypocapnia*) and, therefore, to a rise in hindbrain pH and reduced central chemoreceptor drive, inhibiting the stimulant effect of the hypoxic drive.

With maintained exposure to the hypoxic environment, the inhibition of central chemoreceptor drive diminishes over the next several days. Most rapidly, there is over 1–2 days' diffusion of excess bicarbonate ions out of the interstitial fluid around the central chemoreceptors that reduces buffering of interstitial protons. Over the next 2–3 days, renal bicarbonate excretion amplifies this process and restores central pH and respiratory drive to normal despite the maintained hypocapnia, although arterial pH remains slightly more alkaline than normal. As a result of these adjustments, minute ventilation rises progressively over the first week of hypoxic exposure, with an associated progressive increase in work capacity that is due both to the increased inspired air volume and to the fact that the enhanced ventilation has reduced alveolar $PCO_2$ further and, therefore, the oxygen tension of alveolar air rises. At very high altitudes, the decrease in air density may also contribute to increased capacity for maximum ventilation.

## Haematological changes

Over the first few days of exposure to hypoxia, haematological changes increase the capacity of the red blood cell pool to deliver oxygen. The alkalosis produced by hypocapnia increases red cell expression of 2,3-diphosphglycerate (DPG), which shifts the haemoglobin dissociation curve to the right and increases oxygen unloading in the systemic capillaries (Fig. 12.3). Simultaneously, erythropoietin release from the renal medulla in response to hypoxia stimulates red cell production, so that haematocrit rises progressively over the ensuing several weeks.

## ALTITUDE AND WORK CAPACITY

### Benefits of adaptation for exercise capacity at high altitude

The spectrum of compensatory processes means that fully acclimated individuals have vastly better capacities for work than when they first arrive at altitude. They are, however, still not able to achieve workloads identical to

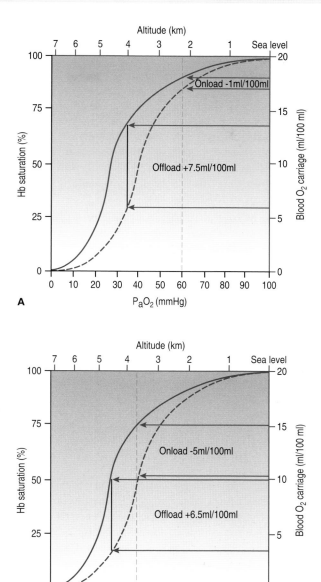

**Figure 12.3** Effect of altitude on the efficiency of DPG expression as an aid to oxygen delivery. Note that the values for PaO$_2$ represent those occurring at the respective altitudes before any compensation. (a) At altitude 2200 m (PaO$_2$ 60 mmHg) there is a doubling of oxygen offloading, while onloading is virtually unaffected. The net tissue gain is 6.5 ml oxygen/100 ml blood. (b) At altitude 3500 m (PaO$_2$ 40 mmHg), by contrast, the improved offloading is almost obviated by reduced onloading. The net tissue gain now is only 1.5 ml oxygen/ 100 ml blood.

those that were possible at sea level. The compensations that occur cannot overcome fully the reduced haemoglobin saturation imposed by a low $PaO_2$ and, in addition, the adaptive processes themselves impose some limits of circulatory efficiency. One problem is that increased haematocrit increases blood viscosity and so increases cardiac workload for a given cardiac output. In addition, the rightwards shift of the haemoglobin dissociation curve induced by DPG has the effect of, under moderate-to-severely hypoxic conditions, reducing pulmonary loading of oxygen as well as increasing the unloading process (Fig. 12.3). Finally, since even slight alkalosis shifts the dissociation curve to the left, the profound hypocapnia seen in fully acclimated individuals may actually reverse the effect of DPG and reduce capillary oxygen unloading.

For athletes who live at low altitudes, a period of acclimation is obviously essential if they are to compete effectively at higher altitudes but, even then, the limits to adaptation described above are likely to restrict their performance. The same limitations are not evident to the same extent in natives of high altitude communities, who appear to possess cardiorespiratory systems that are better adapted to hypoxia. It remains uncertain to what extent these differences from low-level residents are genetically determined and to what extent they are developed during childhood.

## Benefits of adaptation for exercise capacity at low altitude

The greatest significance for athletic performance of adaptations to high altitude is its potential effect on performance at low altitude. Here, the positive effects on oxygen delivery of DPG and raised haematocrit can be exploited without interference from reduced ambient oxygen availability or hypocapnia. This scenario has led to training at altitude being adopted as a routine component of preparation for competition of many athletes. Unfortunately, the value of this strategy is limited by the reduced intensity of training that is possible under hypoxic conditions. More convincing results have been obtained by allowing training to be carried out at low altitude and stimulating the haematological adaptations by exposure to a hypoxic environment overnight (Hendricksenn & Meeuwsen 2003).

The potential advantages for performance of adaptations to hypoxia have led to the administration of synthetic erythropoietin in order to increase haematocrit. Leaving aside the illegality, 'blood doping' with erythropoietin carries with it very substantial risks. The normal response to hypoxia incorporates both increased red cell mass and increased oxygen carriage efficiency through DPG expression. The red cells produced in response to erythropoietin do not have up-regulated DPG and so, in order to achieve a given increment in tissue oxygen delivery, there needs to be a much greater increment in red cell mass. In consequence, athletes who have taken erythropoietin may have haematocrits of the order of 70%, with massively elevated cardiac workload and a significant risk of cardiac events during exercise, as well as increased risk of venous thrombosis due to red cell clumping (see Chapter 5, p. 55).

## PROBLEMS WITH EXPOSURE TO ALTITUDE

### Implications of temperature

Even with ascents that are insufficient to produce significant hypoxia, the effect of altitude on environmental temperature needs to be borne in mind. With every 200 m (660 ft) rise above sea level, air temperature falls by 1.3° C (2.1° F), so that a simple hill walk to a peak standing 1500 m (4900 ft) means exposure to temperatures about 10° C below that at the base. Since increased altitude is also almost inevitably accompanied by greater wind chill and less shelter, hypothermia is an ever-present danger even in moderate climates.

### Dehydration

The progressive temperature fall not only has direct implications for thermo-regulation, but also greatly affects water balance. As air temperature falls, the air becomes progressively drier, so that at 0° C (32° F) saturated water vapour pressure is only around 30% of its value at 20° C (68° F). When this air is inspired, its temperature rises to that of the body and additional water is lost from the airway mucosa in order to saturate it. Ascent to any altitude, therefore, necessarily involves increased water loss. The extent of this must be proportional to the ventilatory volume, so it becomes an increasing prob-lem with increased exercise intensity and especially when the altitude is sufficient for activation of hypoxic respiratory drive. Respiratory dehydra-tion has a powerful enhancing effect on the susceptibility of an individual to hypothermia, since substantial amounts of body heat are lost in warming cold inspired air, while the depletion of plasma volume potentially limits exercise capacity.

### HANDY HINTS

It is often difficult to assess someone's core temperature in the field. Peripheral vasoconstriction may lead to the skin being extremely cold regardless of internal temperature; oral temperature may be inaccurate because of heat loss through the cheeks and because normal oral thermometers cannot register temperatures below around 35°C (95°F).

Estimating the likely extent of hypothermia in a subject and knowing the implica-tions can be helped by considering four critical body core temperatures. At around 34°C (93°F), the heat-producing process of shivering becomes so intense that large

numbers of motor units contract simultaneously. This makes it impossible to under-take fine movements like unfolding a map or adjusting skis. Around 33°C (91.5°F), the limbs are so cold that peripheral axonal conduction is impaired. As a result, heat production through shivering ceases and cutaneous vasoconstriction is inhibited, leading to more rapid heat loss. At this temperature, cerebral metabolism also begins to slow, with confusion and disorientation. At 31°C (90°F), cerebral function is too inefficient to maintain consciousness, so the subject collapses. Finally, at around 27°C (81°F), the pumps that drive cardiac action potentials stop working and car-diac arrest occurs.

The first step in rewarming any hypothermic person is to prevent further heat loss by use of wind–resistant blankets. The next stage has to take into account both the circumstances of cooling and the effects of hypothermia on circulatory reflex control. Individuals who slowly become hypothermic on a hill walk will have low stores of metabolic substrates and may be unable to rewarm themselves spontane-ously, while people who fall into cold water are likely to have cooled down so quickly that their metabolic status is still intact. In either case, if core temperature is below 34°C (93°F) there will be impaired baroreflex function because of reduced sympathetic nerve conduction. To maintain adequate cerebral perfusion, a near–horizontal posture needs to be maintained during rescue and transport.

Finally, if active rewarming outside a clinical setting is necessary, then the circula-tory implications need to be borne in mind. Radiative heat applied to the limbs will initially warm the skin and the resultant inhibition of cutaneous cold receptor activ-ity may lead to withdrawal of sympathetic vasoconstrictor tone and increased limb blood flow. Since the entire tissue of the limbs is hypothermic, the effect may be to cool down venous return to the extent that there is actually a further fall in body temperature before rewarming begins. This may have deleterious effects if the initial core temperature is just above one of the critical values listed – for example, by leading to a deterioration of consciousness that impairs mobility. More efficient rewarming can be achieved by use of a warm bath or by hot water bottles applied only to the trunk.

## Acute mountain sickness

Individuals who ascend rapidly to altitudes around 3000 m (9800 ft) fre-quently suffer from a syndrome termed *acute mountain sickness*, which involves nausea, headache and fatigue, among other symptoms. These symptoms usually appear within 1 or 2 h of ascent and usually disappear over the next several days as acclimation occurs. Several factors may be involved in genesis of acute mountain sickness. Significant dehydration often occurs, because hypoxia and the alkalosis that follows respiratory stim-ulation appear to inhibit thirst and so exaggerate the increased respiratory water loss associated with altitude. This dehydration probably plays a part in the headache by tightening the connective tissue strands that support the brain. Alkalosis seems also to be a key factor in the other symptoms, since most people can prevent acute mountain sickness except at extreme altitudes by dosing themselves with a carbonic anhydrase inhibitor before ascent.

## Pulmonary oedema

A small number of individuals show a more serious acute response to the same levels of ascent that induce acute mountain sickness. In these people, there is damage to the pulmonary capillary wall so that plasma leaks into the lung interstitium and may enter the alveoli. The precise mechanisms that underlie this *high-altitude pulmonary oedema* are not fully understood, but it almost certainly involves generation of high intracapillary pressures in response to hypoxia. Superficially, this seems counterintuitive. You will remember from Chapter 8 (pp. 94) that capillary hydrostatic pressure in the lung is normally well below the plasma oncotic pressure, so that there is a good safety margin to ensure no fluid extravasation. We also saw in Chapter 8 (pp. 96) that the pulmonary arteriolar smooth muscle possesses hypoxia receptors that induce vasoconstriction in response to reduced alveolar $PO_2$. In theory, therefore, breathing hypoxic air should cause generalized pulmonary vasoconstriction which, while it will elevate pulmonary arterial pressure, will reduce capillary hydrostatic pressure.

In practice, the likely explanation is that, in the susceptible individuals that suffer high altitude pulmonary oedema, not all areas of the pulmonary arteriolar bed respond equally strongly to the vasoconstrictor effect of hypoxia. Under these circumstances, a disproportionate volume of right cardiac output is directed through the least constricted vessels exposing the capillaries in these areas to an intravascular pressure close to pulmonary arterial pressure (West 2004).

---

## Case history

A class of 11–12-year-old students from a seaside Irish town travelled on an exchange trip to an alpine village in Switzerland (altitude 2800 m, 9100 ft). On the second day of the visit, one of the students (Kevin B) reported sick, with breathlessness and bluish lips and face. His parents were contacted and he was flown home, although his symptoms had disappeared by the time he had reached the Swiss airport. When the supervising teacher met Kevin's parents they said that he has always had 'a heart murmur' and that medical advice had been for him to avoid strenuous activities, although nobody had mentioned any problems with high altitude. The school doctor examined him, confirmed the presence of a murmur and recorded his resting heart rate as 90 and his blood pressure as 130/60.

# Discussion

Breathlessness, or dyspnoea, is a subjective feeling caused by inadequate pulmonary gas exchange activating chemoreceptors. These might be central $CO_2$ receptors responding to hypercapnia or peripheral hypoxia receptors responding to inadequate oxygenation of arterial blood or to plasma-borne protons. In either case, the sensation of breathlessness is due partly to inputs from these receptors and partly to the respiratory muscle fatigue that results from increased respiratory work. Breathlessness associated with acute ascent to a higher altitude automatically suggests hypoxia rather than acidosis or hypercapnia and this is consistent with the fact that Kevin's lips were bluish. Blue colouration of the mucous membranes or skin, known as cyanosis, reflects the presence in arterial blood of more than 5 g/100 ml of deoxygenated haemoglobin. Thus, cyanosis usually indicates inefficient pulmonary uptake of oxygen. In individuals who have very high haematocrits, on the other hand, it is sometimes possible to see cyanosis in the presence of normal pulmonary oxygenation, because at high rates of pulmonary blood flow there is not enough time to saturate the extra haemoglobin molecules.

Many people have detectable heart murmurs and the cause of these is not always obvious without investigations. From the discussions in Chapter 3 (pp. 24) you will remember that the only criterion for generation of a murmur is the presence of turbulent flow at some time during the cardiac cycle. In most cases, the structural distortion that produces this turbulent flow is a minor one that does not interfere with exercise but, unless the extent of the abnormality has been clarified, you cannot be sure of this. Possible causes of turbulence are valvular stenosis, valvular incompetence or a shunt that allows a proportion of stroke volume to be ejected through a narrow orifice at high velocity.

A resting heart rate of 90 beats/min is high, but not abnormal for a growing child. Similarly, a diastolic pressure of 60 mmHg is within the normal range. However, the combination of these values with a systolic pressure as high as 130 is unexpected. With a cardiac interval of about 700 ms you would expect a resting pulse pressure of around 40 mmHg or slightly below. Kevin's pulse pressure was 70 mmHg, which suggests that stroke volume was substantially elevated above normal. The murmur cannot have been due to atrioventricular valve stenosis or incompetence, semilunar valve stenosis or an inter-atrial or an inter-ventricular shunt, because these would all reduce cardiac ejection and stroke volume. The alternatives are, therefore, semilunar incompetence, with diastolic backflow, or a shunt between the aorta and a low-pressure site. By far the most common shunt of this type in young people is a patent ductus arteriosus.

Would one of these alternatives be able to explain Kevin's breathlessness at altitude? We know that a patent ductus arteriosus will normally shunt blood from aorta to pulmonary artery. We know also that hypoxia elevates pulmonary vascular resistance; if this elevation were large enough pulmonary arterial pressure might exceed aortic pressure, reversing the shunt and resulting in reduced pulmonary blood flow and reduced oxygen uptake. So this would be consistent with Kevin's case, but is it realistic? The degree of hypoxia experienced at 2800 m will approximately double pulmonary blood pressure which, assuming a normal pulmonary pressure of around 25/8 mmHg, would still be lower than Kevin's systemic blood pressure. However, the left–right shunting through a patent ductus arteriosus begins at birth, so Kevin's pulmonary vasculature had been exposed to 12 years of elevated pressure. Arteries and arterioles respond to chronically increased transmural pressure with muscular hypertrophy and this encroaches on the vascular lumen; therefore, Kevin's absolute pulmonary vascular resistance and pulmonary blood pressure would be much higher than normal. Under these circumstances, even a relatively small further increase in pulmonary pressure may reverse the ductus shunt and reduce pulmonary perfusion.

## Pulmonary hypertension

Chronic hypoxia also has other disadvantageous consequences that are seen in long-term residents and, in particular, in individuals who have been born at high altitude. The pulmonary vasoconstrictor effect of hypoxia generates an increased afterload for the right ventricle leading to myocardial hypertrophy and the possibility of right heart failure because of inadequate coronary vascularization (see Chapter 8, p. 95). In addition, the relatively low $PaO_2$ results in reduced efficiency of ductus arteriosus closure after birth (see Chapter 8, p. 102), so that a relatively large number of native highland children have some residual shunting between pulmonary and systemic circulations, which further increases pulmonary afterload.

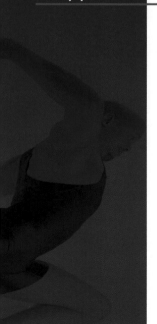

### Key points

As one ascends above sea level, exercise capacity becomes increasingly limited by ventilatory capacity to deliver oxygen to the bloodstream.

The threshold altitude for limiting $\dot{V}O_{2max}$ in sedentary individuals is around 1500 m (5000 ft), but a considerably lower ascent is needed to impair performance in trained athletes with higher cardiac outputs.

Short-term compensations to improve exercise capacity at altitude include increased ventilation triggered by peripheral hypoxia receptors and up-regulation of 2,3-DPG expression in erythrocytes. Over a longer timecourse, these are augmented by increased red cell mass.

The effects of hypoxia can be utilized to improve exercise performance at lower altitudes, with better results produced by exposure to a hypoxic environment for part of the day, but with training performed at a low altitude.

Exposure to altitude is associated with increased risk of dehydration and hypothermia, as well as with the consequences of hypoxia and alkalosis.

## References

Hendriksenn IJ, Meeuwsen T 2003 The effect of intermittent training in hypobaric hypoxia on sea-level exercise: a cross-over study in humans. European Journal of Applied Physiology 88: 396–403.

Johnson RL, Grover RF, DeGraff AC 1994 Effects of high altitude and training on oxygen transport and exercise performance. In: Fletcher GF (ed.) Cardiovascular response to exercise. Futura Publishing Co, Mt Kisco, NY, pp. 223–252.

West JB 2004 The physiologic basis of high-altitude diseases. Annals of Internal Medicine 141: 789–800.

## Further reading

Sallis R, Chassay CM 1999 Recognizing and treating common cold-induced injury in outdoor sports. Medicine and Science in Sports and Exercise 31: 1367–1373.

Schmidt W, Heinicke K, Rojas J et al 2002 Blood volume and hemoglobin mass in endurance athletes from moderate altitude. Medicine and Science in Sports and Exercise 34: 1934–1940.

### Questions for revision

- Using quantitative data, explain the effects on atmospheric and arterial oxygen concentrations of ascent to altitude.

- Compare and contrast the effects on exercise capacity of ascent to 2000 m (6700 ft) and 2500 m (8400 ft) for a period of 4 days.

- What factors reduce maximal work capacity in a resident at high altitude, relative to the same individual's performance at sea level?

- Discuss the benefits and limitations of high-altitude training.

- What factors need to be considered when treating a victim of high-altitude-related hypothermia?

# Chapter questions

Chapter 2

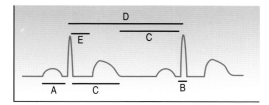

Which of the labelled time intervals on the ECG record shown above:

1. Has a lower normal limit of 120 ms?
2. Is 500 ms in a person with a heart rate of 120 beats/min?
3. Marks the duration of the endocardial ventricular refractory period?
4. Is shortened by increasing the velocity of action potential conduction through the myocardial syncytium?
5. Indicates the time available for ventricular filling?
6. Is never longer than 80 ms in a normal heart?

Chapter 3

1. The maximum heart rate that could in theory be achieved by an obese 20-year-old individual is:

    A. 220 beats/min
    B. 200 beats/min
    C. 190 beats/min
    D. 180 beats/min
    E. 170 beats/min

2. During exercise, ventricular filling increases. Factors that contribute to this include:

    A. Increased intrathoracic pressure
    B. Increased ventricular contractility
    C. Increased heart rate

D. Increased atrial contractility

E. All of the above

3. During moderate exercise, cardiac output rises due to increases in both heart rate and stroke volume, but stroke volume peaks at a workload that is significantly below maximum work capacity and further increase of cardiac output is due solely to heart rate elevation. Factors that limit the rise in stroke volume include all of the following EXCEPT:

A. Myocardial calcium channel cycle time

B. Pericardial stiffness

C. Limited catecholamine secretion

D. Ventricular stiffness

E. Ventricular afterload

4. The second heart sound:

A. Marks the end of ventricular contraction

B. Denotes the end of systolic ejection

C. Coincides with the end of the T wave

D. Is prolonged in the presence of A/V valvular incompetence

E. All of the above

5. $CO_2$ production is measured in an exercising subject, in order to calculate cardiac output by the Fick principle. The values obtained are:

$$\text{Arterial } CO_2 - 46 \text{ ml}/100 \text{ ml}$$

$$\text{Venous } CO_2 - 50 \text{ ml}/100 \text{ ml}$$

$$\text{Whole}-\text{body } CO_2 \text{ production} - 600 \text{ ml}/100 \text{ min}$$

Cardiac output is, therefore:

A. 4 l/min

B. 6 l/min

C. 10 l/min

D. 15 l/min

E. 24 l/min

## Chapter 4

1. The elevation of systolic blood pressure caused by sympathetic nervous system activation involves:

A. Increased cardiac contractility

B. Shortened QRS duration

C. Reduced aortic compliance

D. Reduced venous capacity

E. All of the above

2. A subject has a resting heart rate of 66 beats/min and a blood pressure of 114/60 mmHg. Her mean arterial blood pressure is, therefore:

A. 78 mmHg

B. 82 mmHg

C. 87 mmHg

D. 92 mmHg

E. 96 mmHg

3. Routine measurement of blood pressure by auscultation involves detection of Korotkow sounds during inflation of an occlusive cuff around the arm. These sounds are caused by:

A. Turbulent flow in the segment of artery just downstream of the cuff

B. Turbulent flow in the segment of artery compressed by the cuff

C. Collision of blood with the upstream margin of the cuff

D. Turbulent flow in the segment of artery just upstream of the cuff

E. Intermittency of blood flow due to the occlusive pressure being greater than DBP

4. Arterial pulse pressure:

A. Is increased if peripheral resistance falls while stroke volume and heart rate remain constant

B. Is reduced if peripheral resistance falls while stroke volume and heart rate remain constant

C. Is unaffected if peripheral resistance falls while stroke volume and heart rate remain constant

D. Is greater in the aorta than in the brachial artery

E. Is directly proportional to heart rate

5. A subject undertook steady treadmill exercise at 70% maximum work capacity. His BP was 160/64 mmHg and his cardiac output as measured by $CO_2$ rebreathing was 16 l/min. His total peripheral resistance was therefore:

A. 0.14 PRU

B. 0.16 PRU

C. 4 PRU

D. 6 PRU

E. 7 PRU

## Chapter 5

1. Laplace's law dictates that, in blood vessels:

A. Wall tension is proportional to the ratio of wall thickness: luminal diameter

B. Small vessels are more likely to rupture with increased wall tension than are large ones

C. Veins are more likely to rupture with increased wall tension than are arteries

D. Critical closing pressure is higher in microcirculatory beds with high sympathetic vasomotor tone

E. The presence of elastin in the aortic wall reduces the rise in wall tension associated with BP elevation

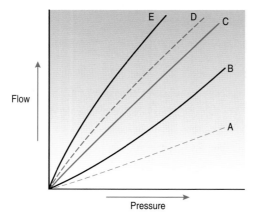

In the above set of curves describing the relationship between pressure gradient and blood flow, which curve represents:

2. Flow through a rigid tube

3. Flow through a relaxed vessel the wall of which contains large amounts of elastin

4. Flow through a relaxed vessel the wall of which contains little elastin

5. Flow through a vessel the wall of which contains large amounts of elastin and in which the smooth muscle is maximally contracted by sympathetic nerve activation

6. Blood viscosity:

A. Is higher in arterial than in arteriolar blood

B. Rises with haematocrit

C. Is lowest in capillaries

D. Falls as flow velocity increases

E. All of the above

## Chapter 6

1. Vasomotion:

A. Occurs only in large arteries

B. Depends on variations in sympathetic vasomotor tone

C. Depends on variations in critical closing pressure

D. Occurs more slowly when tissue metabolic rate rises

E. Occurs typically with a cycle time of 20–30 ms

2. Functional hyperaemia in skeletal muscle during exercise:

A. Is associated with a rise in muscle blood flow of up to 100-fold

B. Commences within a few seconds of the initiation of muscle activity

C. Is due primarily to endothelial factors

D. Involves muscle-derived PGs especially in glycolytic motor units

E. Involves α-adrenoceptor activation by circulating catecholamines

A. kallidin, B. NO, C. potassium ion, D. adrenaline, E. lactate. Which of the dilator mediators listed:

3. Contributes to functional hyperaemia in skin?

4. Contributes to functional hyperaemia by activating guanylate cyclase?

5. Increases capillary permeability as well as causing vasodilation?

6. Is released when blood flow velocity increases?

## Chapter 7

1. The baroreflex response to reduced venous return:

A. Affects peripheral resistance mainly in renal and cutaneous circulations

B. Is more pronounced when arterial compliance is low

C. Results from excitatory inputs from the baroreceptor afferent pathway onto the hindbrain neurons that control sympathetic drive

D. Has minimal effects on skeletal muscle vascular resistance

E. Includes stimulation of vasopressin release

2. During exercise there is a generalized increase in sympathetic vasoconstrictor discharge. However, glomerular filtration is maintained because:

A. Renal sympathetic innervation is only to vessels of the renal medulla

B. Renal sympathetic innervation affects the large arteries but not the microcirculation

C. Sympathetic activation preferentially constricts the afferent renal arterioles

D. Sympathetic activation preferentially constricts the efferent renal arterioles

E. Autoregulation prevents sympathetic activation from reducing renal blood flow

3. During exercise, mean BP is maintained at a higher value than at rest because:

A. The exercise-related sympathetic excitation is so powerful that it overrides the baroreflex

B. The gain of the baroreflex is reduced

C. The operating point of the baroreflex is shifted

D. The baroreflex is not effective when stroke volume is large

E. The BP increase that occurs is a normal baroreflex response to increased venous return

4. The rise in BP associated with exercise is:

   A. Greater with dynamic than with static exercise
   B. Greater with upper-body than with whole-body exercise
   C. In dynamic exercise, due mainly to muscle metaboreceptor activation
   D. More pronounced for DBP than for SBP
   E. Always proportional to the degree of tachycardia

5. During exercise, the increase in coronary blood flow:

   A. Is around fourfold if cardiac output increases fourfold
   B. Involves a change from intermittent to continuous capillary perfusion
   C. Is greater in right than in left ventricle
   D. Is due primarily to β-adrenoreceptor activation
   E. None of the above

6. The elevation of BP during static exercise:

   A. Is due primarily to limb mechanoreceptor activation
   B. Is greatest at maximal workload
   C. Is greater in magnitude for DBP than for SBP
   D. Is minimal unless a large muscle mass is involved
   E. None of the above

---

## Chapter 8

1. The pulmonary ventilation:perfusion ratio:

   A. Is greater than 1.0 throughout the lung, in a supine resting subject
   B. Is less than 1.0 throughout the lung, in a supine resting subject
   C. Is greater than 1.0 in the upper thorax, in a standing resting subject
   D. Is less than 1.0 in the upper thorax, in a standing resting subject
   E. Is 1.0 throughout the lung, in a standing resting subject

2. The pulmonary pressure gradient is only around one-seventh of that in the systemic circulation. As a result:

   A. Pulmonary capillary hydrostatic pressure is similar to intra-alveolar pressure
   B. Cardiac workload is greater in right heart than in the left heart
   C. Cardiac workload rises more in the right than in the left heart when cardiac output increases
   D. Pulmonary wedge pressure can be used as a beat-to-beat index of left ventricular pressure
   E. Right coronary perfusion is continuous rather than intermittent

3. Efficient blood oxygenation during heavy exercise involves:

   A. Mechanical expansion of non-ventilated areas of lung
   B. Dilation of pulmonary arterioles by withdrawal of hypoxia receptor stimulation

C. Elevated systolic pulmonary arterial pressure

D. All of the above

E. None of the above

4. Full $O_2$ saturation of blood can be achieved during moderate exercise without any alterations in ventilation:perfusion matching BECAUSE:

A. At rest, not all the available haemoglobin molecules are fully saturated

B. At rest, the $O_2$ content of the pulmonary capillary plasma is higher than is needed for haemoglobin saturation

C. At rest, $O_2$ concentrations in plasma and alveolar air equilibrate before the plasma has traversed the pulmonary capillary

D. Exercise shifts the haemoglobin dissociation curve to the right

E. Exercise shifts the haemoglobin dissociation curve to the left

5. In the fetal circulation, the entire systemic venous return bypasses the pulmonary circulation BECAUSE:

A. The partition between left and right ventricles is not yet developed

B. The lungs are filled with fluid

C. Local PG secretion causes pulmonary vasoconstriction

D. Low fetal blood oxygenation causes pulmonary vasoconstriction

E. The atrioventricular valves are not yet developed

## Chapter 9

1. Fluid loss due to sweating during exercise:

A. Is associated with loss of around 2.5 g sodium chloride/l sweat in a non-heat acclimatized subject

B. May be up to 5l fluid/h during heavy exercise in a non-heat acclimatized subject

C. Is greater under conditions of low environmental humidity

D. Is more pronounced in children than in adults

E. Is more pronounced in elderly than in young adults

2. Fluid replacement during exercise is facilitated by:

A. Ensuring that the fluid is as cold as possible

B. Ingesting large volumes infrequently

C. Using a hypertonic fluid

D. Using an isotonic fluid

E. Adding small amounts of glucose to the fluid

3. During continuous dynamic exercise, work capacity falls BECAUSE:

A. Increased skin blood flow reduces muscle perfusion

B. Circulating blood volume falls

    C. Blood viscosity rises

    D. Cardiac filling time decreases

    E. All of the above

4. Cardiovascular function during swimming differs from that during running in that:

    A. Sweat is removed from the skin more efficiently

    B. Greater intrathoracic suction increases venous return

    C. The external pressure reduces venous return

    D. The reduced gravitational field increases venous return

    E. Muscle perfusion is a smaller proportion of total cardiac output

5. In adults, the capacity for exercise decreases with age BECAUSE:

    A. Increased cardiac compliance reduces cardiac ejection fraction

    B. Increased resting heart rate reduces heart rate reserve

    C. Reduced heart rate reserve decreases cardiac filling time

    D. Increased aortic compliance reduces the pressor response

    E. Both B and C.

---

## Chapter 10

1. The Valsalva manoeuvre can result in fainting in athletes undertaking heavy resistive exercise. Factors involved in this loss of consciousness include:

    A. Cerebral vasoconstriction due to hypocapnia

    B. Cerebral vasoconstriction due to adrenomedullary stimulation

    C. Plasma volume depletion

    D. All of the above

    E. Both A and B above

2. The recreational drug ecstasy has all of the following effects EXCEPT:

    A. Resetting the hypothalamic thermostat

    B. Reducing skin blood flow

    C. Uncoupling mitochondrial respiration from ATP production

    D. Decreasing thyroid hormone secretion

    E. Stimulating central sympathetic drive

3. Individuals with defects in the RYR1 gene may be at danger during exercise. This is because:

    A. The RYR1 gene controls calcium movement across the muscle cell membrane

    B. The RYR1 gene controls calcium release from the sarcoplasmic reticulum

    C. The RYR1 gene controls calcium movement into vascular smooth muscle

    D. These individuals cannot produce enough muscle contraction to sustain exercise

    E. These individuals cannot produce enough muscle vasodilation to sustain exercise

4. Exertional hyperthermia:

    A. Is most likely in humid environments
    B. Cannot occur so long as plasma volume is not depleted
    C. Is most effectively treated by immersion in chilled water
    D. Results in cessation of exercise before the core temperature becomes dangerously high
    E. All of the above

5. Fluid depletion:

    A. Results in hypotension if blood volume falls by more than 5%
    B. Affects muscle perfusion before it affects other regional beds
    C. Affects renal and intestinal function because of the presence of counter-current loops
    D. Is the basis of the syndrome termed 'heat stroke'
    E. All of the above

## Chapter 11

    A. Heart rate reserve 150 beats/min, cardiac reserve 18 l/min, maximum sweat rate 1.2 l/h, sweat sodium content 45 mmol
    B. Heart rate reserve 120 beats/min, cardiac reserve 18 l/min, maximum sweat rate 1.2 l/h, sweat sodium content 45 mmol
    C. Heart rate reserve 130 beats/min, cardiac reserve 19 l/min, maximum sweat rate 1.5 l/h, sweat sodium content 10 mmol
    D. Heart rate reserve 150 beats/min, cardiac reserve 24 l/min, maximum sweat rate 1.5 l/h, sweat sodium content 10 mmol
    E. Heart rate reserve 120 beats/min, cardiac reserve 24 l/min, maximum sweat rate 1.5 l/h, sweat sodium content 10 mmol
    F. Heart rate reserve 150 beats/min, cardiac reserve 24 l/min, maximum sweat rate 1.5 l/h, sweat sodium content 10 mmol
    G. Heart rate reserve 150 beats/min, cardiac reserve 24 l/min, maximum sweat rate 1.5 l/h, sweat sodium content 45 mmol

In a healthy, 30-year-old subject (resting HR 72 beats/min, resting cardiac output 5.4 l/min), which of the above sets of values best represent the situation:

1. In the sedentary state

2. After dynamic exercise training for 3 weeks

3. After dynamic training for 6 months

4. The earliest detectable cardiovascular adaptation to training is:

    A. A fall in resting heart rate
    B. A rise in haematocrit

C. A rise in plasma volume

D. A decrease in resting stroke volume

E. An increase in resting stroke volume

5. Eccentric cardiac hypertrophy:

   A. Involves increases in both ventricular muscle mass and ventricular chamber volume

   B. Occurs in response to increased afterload

   C. During training, occurs in left heart before it occurs in right heart

   D. Is maximal after around 3 months' training

   E. Is more likely to be associated with cardiac arrhythmias than is concentric hypertrophy

6. Chronic dynamic exercise is thought to reduce the risk of atherogenesis. Probable mechanisms involved include:

   A. Reduced microcirculatory shear stress

   B. Slower endothelial cell turnover

   C. Lower peripheral resistance

   D. Increased sympathetic drive

   E. All of the above

---

## Chapter 12

A. $PaO_2$ 55 mmHg, $PaCO_2$ 30 mmHg, arterial pH 7.40

B. $PaO_2$ 55 mmHg, $PaCO_2$ 30 mmHg, arterial pH 7.45

C. $PaO_2$ 55 mmHg, $PaCO_2$ 35 mmHg, arterial pH 7.65

D. $PaO_2$ 100 mmHg, $PaCO_2$ 40 mmHg, arterial pH 7.40

E. $PaO_2$ 100 mmHg, $PaCO_2$ 40 mmHg, arterial pH 7.35

F. $PaO_2$ 90 mmHg, $PaCO_2$ 50 mmHg, arterial pH 7.35

G. $PaO_2$ 100 mmHg, $PaCO_2$ 50 mmHg, arterial pH 7.35

Which of the above blood gas profiles is most likely to have come from:

1. A resident at sea level, at rest

2. A resident at sea level, at the end of a 5000 m race

3. A resident at sea level, 3 h after ascent to an altitude of 3000 m

4. An individual who has been resident at 3000 m for several days

5. Exercise performance is reduced by altitude more in trained athletes than in sedentary individuals BECAUSE:

   A. Training shifts the haemoglobin saturation curve to the right

   B. Training shifts the haemoglobin saturation curve to the left

   C. The greater cardiac output achieved in athletes reduces pulmonary oxygen uptake

D. The increased haematocrit in athletes increases their cardiac workload

E. Absolute work capacity is reduced by hypoxia

6. A young man collapses during a winter hill walk. He is not shivering and, although he is conscious, he seems confused. This picture is characteristic of deep body temperatures in the range:

   A. 35–36° C

   B. 34–35° C

   C. 32–34° C

   D. 30–32° C

   E. 28–30° C

# Chapter answers

---

## Chapter 2

1. A. The conduction velocity of the AV node results in a PR interval that is always between 120–200 ms in a normal heart.

2. D. A heart rate of 120 beats/min corresponds to two beats every second.

3. C. Since the T wave denotes the period during which ventricular repolarization takes place, the end of this wave corresponds to repolarization of the longest duration action potentials, which are those in the endocardial cells.

4. B. The duration of the QRS complex denotes the time taken for depolarization of the entire ventricular myocardium.

5. F. The AV valves open when ventricular muscle relaxation is complete and close at the beginning of ventricular contraction.

6. B. The normal velocity of impulse propagation through the ventricular syncytium causes depolarization of the whole muscle mass within 50–80 ms. If the time taken for ventricular depolarization is greater than 80 ms, then the velocity of action potential propagation is abnormally slow OR the normal conduction pathway is blocked at some point.

---

## Chapter 3

1. C. For an obese person, the calculated heart rate maximum is (200-age/2) beats/min.

2. D. Release of catecholamines increases contractility of all myocardial cells, but it is only atrial contraction that can contribute to ventricular filling. Other factors that aid filling are decreased intrathoracic pressure during inspiration and muscle pumping causing compression of limb veins. Increased heart rate may increase end-systolic volume, but does not affect ventricular filling.

3. C. Ventricular filling is limited by the increased stiffness of both myocardium and pericardium at high filling volumes and by the fact that the calcium channels that determine ventricular action potential plateau duration have a finite minimum cycle time, so that above a certain heart rate the diastolic filling time is shortened. With exercise modalities that elevate diastolic blood pressure, this rise in afterload also limits ventricular emptying. Sympathetic activation and catecholamine secretion continue to rise proportionately to exercise intensity up to maximum work capacity.

4. B. The second heart sound is due to semilunar valve closure and, therefore, denotes the end of cardiac ejection. The semilunar valves close as soon as the ventricles begin to relax, coincident with the beginning of the T wave.

5. D. Each 100 ml of blood loses (50–46) = 4 ml $CO_2$ as it passes through the lungs. If whole-body $CO_2$ production is 600 ml/min, then the total volume of blood passing through the lungs in this time must be (600/4).100 ml or 15 l/min.

## Chapter 4

1. E. Sympathetic activation increases stroke volume both by increasing cardiac filling (due primarily to mobilizing blood from venous reservoirs) and by increasing cardiac emptying (due to increased myocardial contractility). The effect on peak blood pressure of this larger stroke volume is enhanced by faster ejection by more rapid myocardial depolarization and by reduced aortic distension because of vascular muscle contraction.

2. A. Remember that the formula for calculation of mean blood pressure at rest is DBP + ⅓ PP or (SBP + 2DBP). Only at the high heart rates that occur during heavy exercise, DBP + ⅖ PP, may be slightly more accurate.

3. A. Conversion of laminar to turbulent flow is enhanced by increased velocity of flow and increased vessel diameter. This situation occurs where blood whose flow velocity has been increased by vessel compression under the cuff enters the wider, non-compressed segment immediately downstream. With cuff inflation to pressures between systolic and diastolic pressures, flow is necessarily intermittent. However, with the high flow velocities associated with high cardiac outputs, Korotkow sounds may still be heard when the cuff is inflated to pressures significantly below DBP and flow is continuous.

4. C. Decreased peripheral resistance will reduce DBP. If stroke volume and heart rate remain constant, then the pulse pressure will remain constant. Pulse pressure is inversely proportional to heart rate if all other factors remain unchanged, and is greater in peripheral arteries than in aorta because aortic compliance damps the pressure oscillations.

5. D. Peripheral resistance = mean BP/CO = 96/16 PRU. Remember that the PRU unit varies in magnitude depending on the way in which cardiac output is expressed. Here, the PRU incorporates cardiac output as expressed in l/min. If cardiac output was expressed in ml/min, then peripheral resistance would be 96/16 000 or 0.006 PRU.

## Chapter 5

1. D. When sympathetic tone is high, a greater intravascular pressure is needed to balance the tendency of the vessel wall to contract inwards. Wall tension is proportional to transmural pressure and to the ratio of luminal diameter:wall thickness, so it rises with BP and is higher in large vessels with high intravascular pressures. The elastic properties of the aortic wall make it stretch in response to increased BP; the presence of collagen limits this expansion and the risk of rupture.

2. C.

3. A.

4. B.

5. B.

6. E. Properties A, B and D are a necessary consequence of blood containing a suspension of cellular components. The very low viscosity seen in capillaries is a result of the lubricant that lines the capillary endothelial cells.

## Chapter 6

1. C. Vasomotion describes the process of intermittent opening and closing of metarterioles supplying different areas of a tissue capillary bed. This is due to local oscillations in critical closing pressure dependent on the rate of interstitial metabolite accumulation. The cycle time in a resting tissue is typically of the order of 20–30 s.

2. B. The rapid onset of hyperaemia at the beginning of muscle activity is probably due to liberation of potassium ions from the contracting cells. The subsequent sustained hyperaemia, which may reach 10–20 times resting flow, is due primarily to muscle-derived metabolites, with smaller contributions from endothelium-derived factors, catecholamine-induced β-adrenoreceptor activation and, particularly in oxidative motor units, muscle-derived NO and PGs.

3. A. The process of eccrine sweat secretion liberates into the glandular interstitium both kallidin and the associated vasodilator peptide, bradykinin.

4. B.

5. A. The increased capillary permeability caused by kinin liberation in exocrine glands optimizes the extravasation of water and electrolytes needed for glandular secretion.

6. B. Increased endothelial shear stress results in liberation from the endothelial cells of several vasodilator factors including NO, EDHF and PGs.

## Chapter 7

1. E. Baroreceptor firing inhibits the hindbrain neurons that activate sympathetic vasomotor drive to kidney, digestive tract and skeletal muscle. The low-pressure atrial baroreceptor pathway also inhibits hypothalamic release of vasopressin. As the baroreceptors function by detecting mechanical distortion of the axon endings, arterial baroreceptor discharge varies less with intravascular pressure when the arterial wall is less distensible.

2. D. The kidney is a major source of peripheral resistance elevation during exercise, but this is achieved primarily by increasing arteriolar resistance distal to the glomeruli, so that the effect on filtration of reduced glomerular blood flow is balanced by the increased glomerular capillary hydrostatic pressure.

3. C. Resetting of the operating point is thought to be due to input from the central command. The sustained elevation of BP is useful in maintaining nutritional perfusion to those tissues in which vascular resistance has been increased by the exercise response.

4. B. The more pronounced pressor response to upper-body exercise is due mainly to the greater total peripheral resistance that results from sympathetic vasoconstriction in the inactive muscles of the lower body. BP elevation is greatest during static activity due to input from muscle metaboreceptors and at high static loads the reduction in venous return may lead to a fall in stroke volume and SBP.

5. A. Coronary blood flow rises proportionately to cardiac workload and this is reflected by cardiac output. Since even at rest there is some degree of functional hyperaemia in the coronary circulation, all coronary capillaries are always open. As the left heart produces more work than the right, functional hyperaemia must be greater on the left side. Around 25% of the exercise-induced coronary hyperaemia is due to β-adrenoreceptor activation by sympathetic nerves and circulating adrenaline (epinephrine).

6. E. The pressor response to static exercise is pronounced even with contraction of small muscle groups and is due primarily to metaboreceptor stimulation and central command. Because of the absence of muscle perfusion, peripheral resistance rises in response to the increased sympathetic drive, and so both DBP and SBP increase proportionately. At maximal workloads, the mechanical restriction to venous return often causes a fall in stroke volume sufficient to lower BP slightly.

## Chapter 8

1. C. Although both ventilation and perfusion are lower at the lung apices than the lung bases in a standing individual, blood flow is reduced to a greater extent due to the difficulty in pumping blood against a gravitational head.

2. E. The relatively low right ventricular systolic pressure means that cardiac workload is always lower in right than in left heart and that the right coronary vasculature is not occluded during cardiac contraction. The small pressure loss between pulmonary arteries and veins means that wedge pressure can be used to approximate beat-to-beat left atrial pressure.

3. D. The combination of increased tidal volume, increased right heart stroke volume and pulmonary arteriolar dilatation produces more efficient gas exchange in areas of lung that are either not fully perfused or not fully ventilated at rest.

4. C. Since there is equilibration between air and plasma by the time the plasma has travelled about ⅓ of the length of the pulmonary capillary, cardiac output can rise around threefold before $O_2$ uptake begins to be impaired. Shifts in the haemoglobin curve affect offloading of $O_2$, but have no effect on haemoglobin uptake of $O_2$ at normal $PaO_2$.

5. B. Intrapulmonary fluid compresses the pulmonary vasculature and elevates pulmonary vascular resistance so that blood passes preferentially from the right atrium into the left atrium via the foramen ovale and from the main pulmonary artery to the aorta via the ductus arteriosus.

## Chapter 9

1. A. Sweat in non-heat acclimatized individuals contains around 2.5 g sodium chloride/l and cannot be secreted at rates greater than around 1 l/h. Secretion is less efficient in children and older adults. When relative humidity is low, evaporative heat loss is more efficient and so less sweat is needed to achieve thermal stability.

2. E. Absorption of fluid is enhanced by ingestion of hypotonic fluid containing around 20 g glucose/l. Gastric emptying is slowed if the fluid is very cold or if a large volume is ingested.

3. E. Muscle perfusion is reduced both by diversion of some cardiac output to skin to service thermoregulatory demands and by the progressive fall in plasma volume due primarily to sweating. These factors result in greater encroachment on heart rate reserve, with reduced efficiency of cardiac filling. The rise in heart rate and the increased blood viscosity caused by plasma depletion increase cardiac workload for any given exercise intensity.

4. D. During swimming, neither sweating nor increased skin perfusion is necessary for heat loss. As well, the external pressure and the horizontal posture increase venous return. The net result is enhanced muscle perfusion relative to the situation during terrestrial exercise.

5. C. The age-dependent fall in maximum heart rate reduces capacity to elevate cardiac output, although resting heart rate is not affected by age. Ageing is associated with generalized loss of elastin from tissues, with a consequent decrease in aortic compliance.

## Chapter 10

1. D. The reduction in cerebral perfusion induced by the Valsalva manoeuvre is exaggerated by hypocapnia and by circulating adrenaline (epinephrine), both of which raise cerebral vascular resistance, and by reduced plasma volume associated with voluntary weight reduction.

2. D. Ecstasy increases thyroid hormone release and, therefore, up-regulates basal metabolic rate in chronic users.

3. B. Abnormality of the RYR1 gene causes excessive calcium release from skeletal muscle sarcoplasmic reticulum onto the sarcomeres, with local heat-induced muscle damage and generalized hyperthermia.

4. A. Hyperthermia is more likely when reduced plasma volume jeopardizes sweat production and skin perfusion, but may occur without fluid depletion if the individual is wearing clothing that prevents heat exchange. Highly motivated athletes are sometimes able to continue exercise even in the face of severe hyperthermia. Because of reflex vasoconstrictor responses to skin cooling, immersion in tepid rather than cold water is the more effective treatment for most cases of hyperthermia.

5. C. The countercurrent organization of the microcirculation in renal medulla and intestinal villi means that these areas are especially sensitive to hypoxic damage when blood flow is reduced. Hypotension results from falls in blood volume above around 20% and, in the upright position, cerebral perfusion will be most sensitive to this. The collapse consequent upon plasma volume depletion is termed heat exhaustion to distinguish it from the direct effect of hyperthermia, known as heat stroke.

## Chapter 11

1. B. Age-dependent HR maximum is 190 beats/min, so nominal heart rate reserve = (190–72) = 120 beats/min. A sedentary person can increase cardiac output to around four times the resting value = 22 l/min. Normal maximal sweat secretion is around 1 l/h and normal sweat sodium content is around 50 mmol.

2. C. The increased plasma volume due to training for 3 weeks would be expected to produce a resting bradycardia of up to 10 beats/min, with a small consequent increase in maximum

cardiac output. The expanded blood volume and the associated increase in peripheral aldosterone receptors will increase maximum sweat production and increase sweat duct reabsorption of sodium ion.

3. F. Training for an extended period can be predicted to produce more pronounced resting bradycardia than would occur during short term activity, due to cardiac remodelling. This will lead to a proportionate rise in maximum cardiac output.

4. C. Plasma volume is increased after only one to two training sessions due to aldosterone-mediated sodium and water retention, leading to a fall in haematocrit. Decreased resting heart rate and increased stroke volume are not seen until training has progressed for some weeks.

5. A. The process of cardiac remodelling in response to chronically increased preload occurs initially in right heart and is not complete in left heart until after around 6–9 months of training. Concentric hypertrophy, which occurs in response to increased afterload, results in a greatly thickened ventricular wall that predisposes to endocardial ischaemia and arrhythmias.

6. C. Chronic dynamic exercise leads to reduced peripheral resistance secondary to peripheral angiogenesis, more rapid endothelial turnover and reduced sympathetic gain. All of these adaptations lower blood pressure, which in turn reduces shear stress in the large arteries where flow velocity is high and lowers the risk of endothelial damage.

## Chapter 12

1. D. These values are all normal.

2. E. Although normal gas exchange is maintained so that $PaO_2$ and $PaCO_2$ remain normal, lactate accumulation has slightly lowered blood pH.

3. C. The acute response to hypoxia is increased minute ventilation. This produces hypocapnia and so increases blood pH.

4. B. Acclimatization to a hypoxic environment reduces the inhibitory effect of hypocapnia on respiratory drive and so allows greater minute ventilation. As well, renal acid–base compensations to alkalosis take place. As a result, blood pH falls to a value close to normal despite further ventilation-induced hypocapnia.

5. C. As cardiac output during exercise is higher in athletes, there is correspondingly less time for gas exchange in the pulmonary capillaries and so desaturation occurs more easily in the presence of reduced $P_AO_2$.

6. C. Loss of shivering suggests a core temperature below 34° C and preservation of consciousness suggests that core temperature is above 31° C.

# Index